Being Pregnant Was the Easy Part!

Kathi Pitts

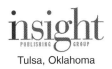
insight
PUBLISHING GROUP

Tulsa, Oklahoma

BEING PREGNANT WAS THE EASY PART!

Being Pregnant Was the Easy Part by Kathi Pitts
Published by Insight Publishing Group
8801 S. Yale, Suite 410
Tulsa, OK 74137
918-493-1718

Unless otherwise noted, Scripture quotations are taken from *Compton's Interactive Bible NIV*. Copyright © 1994, 1995, 1996 SoftKey Multimedia Inc. All Rights Reserved.

Scriptures marked NKJV are taken from *The Holy Bible, New King James Version*, (Nashville, Tennessee: Thomas Nelson, Inc.) 1982.

Scriptures marked NLT are taken from *Holy Bible, New Living Translation*, (Wheaton, IL: Tyndale House Publishers, Inc.) 1996.

ISBN 1-932503-18-8
Library of Congress catalog card number: 2004101668

Printed in the United States of America

Contents

Dedication
Acknowledgements
Foreword
Preface

Chapter One
   A Heritage and a Reward 13
Chapter Two
   God's Way Is Best! 21
Chapter Three
   Parenting: Godly Leadership 29
Chapter Four
   Learning to Love 39
Chapter Five
   Praying for Your Children 51
Chapter Six
   You Are a Cheerleader! 69
Chapter Seven
   Response-Able 87
Chapter Eight
   Rewards and Bribes 97
Chapter Nine
   The Dynamic Duo: Honor and Obedience 105

Chapter Ten

Correction and Discipline 117

Chapter Eleven

Teaching Your Children the Word of God 133

Chapter Twelve

Fearfully and Wonderfully Made 141

Dedication

How could I not dedicate this book to our incredible children?
❧ Meredith and Stephen Michael ☙
You bless your father and I more than you'll ever know.
You're the best—lots of love to you always!

Acknowledgements

Thank you to my husband Michael Pitts. Every day you help me believe in me. Your encouragement and support in this process have truly been invaluable. You have the most incredible heart—I love you.

Thank you to my parents, Jack and Janette Gamble. You taught me to love God and always put Him first. If there is a top ten list of the nicest people in the world, I know the two of you are on it. I love you!

Most importantly to my Father God—how could I be without you?

Foreword

The most valuable gift that could be given to the world is a well-educated, disciplined, mature, visionary child. The future of all nations is hidden in the children of the next generation. Children and youth are the hope of the future and the key to a better world.

Whenever God wanted to change the world or bring change to a nation, He never attacked the present government or the powers that be; He simply used a baby. When the children of Israel were slaves to the Egyptians, God's strategy was not to attack or address the Pharaoh of Egypt directly. He preserved a baby in a basket, and he was destined to change the course of history for both Egypt and Israel. God's ultimate strategy for saving mankind was also through a baby, this one in a manger. This is the ultimate divine strategy! To change the world, we must concentrate on the children.

It is also interesting to note that when Jesus Christ was about to transfer His leadership to the disciple Peter, His instructions were not that Peter was to feed His sheep first. But rather, He said, "Feed my *lambs.*" The priority was on the young ones. The key to our nation's future is our children. When we invest in our children's development, we express the very nature of God.

The greatest role an adult can play in life is that of a parent. Parenting is the most honorable responsibility of our society, but the difficulty is that most people with children know little about parenting!

We take it for granted that when we purchase a product we normally receive a book of instruction called the manual. The manual provides the information and instructions on how to operate and care for the product.

This makes it easier and safer to use the product and minimizes experimentation. In fact, the manual also usually contains the manufacturer's guarantee and warranty.

However, no owner's manual comes with the arrival of a new baby. Parenting is an art that has to be learned and developed. It is a practice that must be taught and transferred. It is sad to say that most parents in today's society have little or no formal training on parenting, and the results of this lack is evident in the quality of the new generations of children in our nations.

Parents need help.

This is why I am so excited about this book, *Being Pregnant Was the Easy Part*. It is a work that is overdue and needed in the marketplace. The profound thoughtfulness hidden in these pages has the potential to start a social revolution that could change the face of our nations if embraced and applied by the reader.

Kathi Pitts, in this work, leaps over complicated philosophies and distills the heart of what it takes to be an effective and efficient parent. The technical skills are balanced by the warm precepts of love, sensitivity, and compassion necessary for parenting. In this work, we also learn the difference between loving discipline and abuse. The spiritual foundations on which her premises are built provide the sound perspective that gives us a sense of confidence in cultivating and incubating the next generation. This book makes parenting fun!

I believe this book will be to parenting what your manual is to your product. It's a handbook on the oldest profession in the world—parenting. Open these pages and explore the joys of parenting your godly heritage. The future depends on it! Do it for the sake of the unborn, and shoot an arrow from your quiver into the future of the world. It's your greatest investment.

DR. MYLES E. MUNROE
Nassau, Bahamas

Preface

Shortly after becoming the mother of two incredible children, *stress* set in. As much as I loved my two little blessings, I started asking God if He would take them back! I felt completely overwhelmed by the whole parenting thing!

I really thought I would be great at it; after all, everyone *else's* kids loved me. As a teenager, I was the neighborhood babysitter. I loved kids. Patience and understanding oozed from my pores. Yet I felt like a complete failure most of the time.

I read all those Scriptures telling me how blessed I was supposed to be and that these darlings were supposed to be some kind of reward to me, but I just wasn't seeing it. My idea of a blessing was stumbling on a great sale at the mall, and a reward was something you celebrated and set out on display so everyone would admire it and congratulate you.

I never imagined a blessing in the form of my children. Some days I even pictured setting my children on the curb with a sign that said, *"For Sale—Best Offer."* Of course I would never *really* have done this, but I must admit, the thought was fun.

When I finally reached my frustration limit, I seriously talked to God about the situation. This book is what happened when I really started listening to the leading of the Holy Spirit—He started answering me! I hope that you will find answers, encouragement, and strength as you read.

The Kingdom of God started with our heavenly Father sowing His seed into the earth. It continues with our seed. The enemy would love nothing more than to keep parents exhausted and frustrated. If parents are exhausted we can't parent from a place of strength and confidence.

I still have moments of frustration and exhaustion, but I don't live there anymore. And you don't have to either! I pray that this book will help you allow the Word of God to teach you to parent your seed. They are the future—they are the Kingdom!

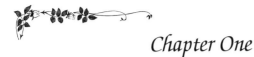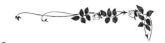

Chapter One

A Heritage and a Reward

Psalm 127:3-5 (NLT) says,

Children are a gift from the Lord; they are a reward from him. Children born to a young man are like sharp arrows in a warrior's hands. How happy is the man whose quiver is full of them! He will not be put to shame when he confronts his accusers at the city gates.

"A reward? My children are a *reward*? What did I do to earn this kind of reward?" Have you asked yourself these questions more often than you'd care to admit? Yet, this is exactly what your children are—*your reward*! The Scripture above tells us that not only are they our reward, they are part of our heritage or inheritance.

If you received a phone call tomorrow telling you that someone in your distant family or a long, lost acquaintance died and left you something as an inheritance, you would be excited. You'd be curious about what this inheritance might be, and you'd be eager to see if it would turn out to be anything of substance. You would talk about it all the time, to yourself and to anyone else who would listen. Your focus would be on discovering what this inheritance was.

Your children are not an inheritance from a person but from the Creator of everything! And what you put in them will continue on beyond their natural lives and into your grandchildren and even great-grandchildren. Jack Hayford said it this way: "Your children are the message you will send to a time you will not see." We should be very excited about this kind of heritage!

We don't have to wonder whether this inheritance, which was sent straight from God, will turn out to be substantial or valuable. The only mystery involved in this inheritance is uncovering and revealing the exact and complete value and purpose of it.

Fearfully and Wonderfully Made

Psalm 139:13-16 says,

For you created my inmost being; you knit me together in my mother's womb. I praise you because I am fearfully and wonderfully made; your works are wonderful, I know that full well. My frame was not hidden from you when I was made in the secret place. When I was woven together in the depths of the earth, your eyes saw my unformed body. All the days ordained for me were written in your book before one of them came to be.

Nothing God creates is without purpose. Every glorious creation of His has an intended use in His Kingdom, and this includes you and your children. This principle of the Kingdom often gets lost in the ugly world in which we live.

Many people, children included, are hurting—desperately hurting. Sin always distorts God's purposes. It disguises them and buries them so you can't see or understand them. Yet God ultimately has a purpose for every person. We learn how to uncover purpose when we turn our hearts and minds to the truth in the Bible.

How is this relevant to the subject of this book? Easy—your children are sent here wrapped up in purpose. You as a parent have the responsibility of helping your children discover and uncover their God-given purpose.

In Psalm 139:14, David writes that he was *"fearfully and wonderfully"* made. The word *fearfully* here means, "with reverence, carefully, with awe." For both of my children's first birthdays, I wanted to make their birthday cakes with my own hands. I wanted them to be special— something just from me. I planned carefully what I would need and how I would make them. These cakes were going to be different from any I had made before; there was something special attached to their creation. I took my time putting them together, painstakingly decorating them so they would be just as I had envisioned them. My attitude toward making these cakes was different.

God is that way every time He creates a life. He does it with reverence and awe. Every life is something special to Him. He doesn't throw lives together like a cheeseburger at a fast food restaurant but carefully puts them together according to His master plan.

The word *wonderfully* means, "to distinguish, put a difference in, separate, set apart." Your child's life is not based on some giant procedural manual or generic, heavenly kid mold. You see, God not only takes His time creating your child's life, He distinguishes it from every other life He has created by giving it its own purpose—its own reason for existence. Before your child was born and drew his first breath, his days were numbered and ordained by the Lord. It was settled in heaven. We'll talk more about how we help discover our children's purposes later in the book.

What Does God Say About Children?

God says your children are a reward and the person with them is blessed. However, if your child is not being a blessing to you and others, then some changes might be in order.

Your children *really are* blessings. However, think of this: if you asked God for a car and He blessed you

Your children really are blessings.

with one but you failed to care for that car as you should, eventually it would feel like a curse and not a blessing. It would break

down at all the most inappropriate times and cost you more than you can imagine to repair. In short, it will eventually cease to serve its purpose.

Likewise, if you fail to nurture and care for your children, your blessing will cost you more than you could ever imagine. Your children will break down and fail to fulfill their purpose. And we've all met them, these *unnurtured* children. It's not their fault. Yet God wants your child—every child—to be a blessing to you and to everyone around them.

You must begin to see and understand your child as God does. Your child is precious to God and to His Kingdom. Jesus said in Matthew 18 that to enter heaven, you must first become as a little child, and that if you accept or receive a little child in His name, you accept or receive Him. But if you offend one of His little ones, you might as well tie a huge stone around your neck, jump into the ocean, and drown!

That's pretty clear and direct to me. This Scripture is talking about salvation, but it's interesting that Jesus used a precious little child as His object lesson. God obviously does not tolerate offending those who have just come to know Him any more than He tolerates someone hurting or offending a small child.

In Matthew 19:13-15 we again see God's attitude toward children displayed. Here we find people bringing their children to Jesus so He can pray for them. His disciples tell the parents to go away. I can just hear them say, "He doesn't have time for these kids! Go away!" But Jesus rebukes them and says, "Don't you understand? The Kingdom of God belongs to them too." In Mark's account of this event, Jesus not only corrected His disciples for sending the children away but also was *"much displeased"* (KJV) and *"indignant"* (NIV) with them for doing so.

Unfortunately, society at large and many of its individuals offend children daily by robbing them of their innocence. Their wide-eyed wonder, curiosity, and natural ability to believe the impossible is stolen from them before they even realize the miracle of it. We've even come to the point where our children are destroying each other!

We could blame the media and its blatant use of sex and violence. We could also blame the drug dealers and gangbangers. We could blame those who promote pornography. What about video games, the Internet, lack of parental involvement, or the general "me first" attitude so prevalent in today's culture? All of these are contributors, but they are not the root of the problem.

The largest offense thrust upon the children of our society is a lack of God in their lives. We have relegated God to Sunday mornings and sweet old ladies. Most children—not to mention countless adults—don't know even the most basic of Bible stories. We've taught them to believe in nothing greater than humanity.

In essence, we have done exactly what the disciples did in Matthew 19, Mark 10, and Luke 18—we have sent the children away from the only Person who can give their lives true value and meaning. We seem to have forgotten to bring our children to Him. Remember the old song, "Jesus loves the little children, all the children of the world. Red, and yellow, black, and white, they are precious in His sight. Jesus loves the little children of the world." Your children are precious and valuable to God.

Psalm 128:1, 3b says, *"Blessed are all who fear the LORD, who walk in his ways.... Your sons will be like olive shoots around your table."* A few years ago as I read this Scripture, I stopped and asked myself, "Olive shoots? Why olive shoots?" As I searched, I discovered what an integral role the olive tree and its fruit played in the culture of the time. They ate the olives, but even more importantly, they depended on the oil from the olive for cooking, heating, lighting, and medicinal purposes. If you owned an olive orchard, you were considered to be wealthy and an important part of your community.

Before they could harvest the olive oil, they first had to grow some good fruit. If an olive shoot is left untended or not pruned, it will usually survive; olive plants are hardy and can often be found growing in the crevices of rocks and other seemingly hostile environments. The question is not one of survival as much as it is one of thriving.

Untended olive shoots grow into a short prickly shrub with long, hard, useless fruit. But if that tender olive shoot is nurtured and pruned, it will grow into a tree that can reach heights of thirty feet, and it will produce good fruit—rich, full, ripe olives that bring prosperity to its owner. These olives will provide oil for baking bread, heating homes, lighting lamps, and healing wounds.

Our children are like these olive shoots—full of potential that's waiting to manifest fruit. If we tend them properly, nurture, and instruct them according to the truths found in the Bible, they will grow into trees instead of scrub bushes. They'll be children full of good fruit.

In the Scriptures, oil is symbolic for the anointing of God. God's anointing sets us apart and empowers us as His people here on the earth. The Scripture from Psalm 128 is a promise that the fruit these mature "olive shoots"—our children—produce will be full of the anointing. This anointing will set them apart from all others. The warmth of God's anointing in their lives will draw those who are out in the cold and hungry into the house of God. With this empowering anointing, they will light a path for those who stumble in the darkness and bring healing to all those who are wounded and dying.

> *Our children are like these olive shoots—full of potential that's waiting to manifest fruit.*

God intends for your children to bring healing and restoration to all those with whom they come in contact. He intends for them to be mighty in *their* land. When they go to school, soccer practice, or karate lessons, they can impact lives—because you chose to delight in following the commands of God. This is the wonderful posterity you can leave for the world and the Kingdom of God: strong, tall, fruit-bearing olive trees—godly children.

When we choose to see our children as God sees them and we set an example of obeying Him, our children will grow up to experience His blessing and His power; they will be blessed and they will be a blessing to us and others. Psalm 112:1,2 says it very well: *"Praise the Lord! Blessed is the man who fears the Lord, who delights greatly in his commandments. His descendants will be mighty on earth; the generation of the upright will be blessed."*

It's important that we begin to look at our children with new attitudes. Look at them through the eyes of God, through the eyes of faith—see them for their potential. God gave them to us as part of our inheritance. They are precious and valuable. God wants them to be mighty, to be part of a godly generation that is righteous and blessed.

Our task is to work together with God to help them discover their purposes and walk out their God-given destiny.

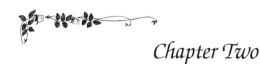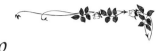

Chapter Two

God's Way Is Best!

Polly Berrien Berends states, "The *real parents* of our children are the ideas that govern us," in her book *Gently Lead*. In other words, the ideas and philosophies by which we live our lives often influence our children more than our conscious parenting techniques. They learn from some combination of what we say and what we actually do, making it vitally important that we live our own lives in a godly manner, based on the Word, so that the ideas that govern us transfer to our children.

The Bible is full of instruction on how to live, and one of my favorites is Psalm 1:1,2 which says,

> *Blessed is the man who does not walk in the counsel of the wicked or stand in the way of sinners or sit in the seat of mockers. But his delight is in the law of the LORD, and on his law he meditates day and night.*

The word *blessed* here is actually the Hebrew word *'esher*, and it means, "to be happy." The root of *'esher* is the Hebrew word *ashar*, which literally means, "to be straight, level, and right." Figuratively, this word can mean, "to move forward, honest, prosper, guide."

So the person who chooses to follow after the law of God will find himself happy because he is on a straight, level path that is right or righteous. The counsel of God will propel you forward and not backward, keep you honest and prosperous, and be a light to your path.

For our own sake as well as for that of our children, we must delight in God's Word and ways every day and in every way. Many of men's philosophies and counsels are flawed, and some of the solutions we find in them are at best temporary—if they work at all. These ways might *seem* right—they might seem like a logical way to raise your children—but the Word tells us that there is a way that seems right but actually leads to death (See Proverbs 14:12 and 16:25.). If we solely depend on men's philosophies we have succumbed to the spirit of the age and it will bring nothing but destruction.

God has made us stewards over our children, but He is sovereign and we must recognize His sovereignty as it relates to our children. Solomon, in his wisdom, knew that God was the real builder of the temple and not him. He penned Psalm 127:1 as the temple he so painstakingly had worked to build was being completed.

Psalm 127:1, 3-5 says,

Unless the LORD builds the house, its builders labor in vain…. Sons are a heritage from the LORD, children a reward from him. Like arrows in the hands of a warrior are sons born in one's youth. Blessed is the man whose quiver is full of them. They will not be put to shame when they contend with their enemies in the gate.

Solomon knew that all of his labor would be in vain if he didn't acknowledge God. If God wasn't in it, it would just be a pretty building. While Solomon was doing the physical work here on the earth, there was a spiritual work going on in the heavens—a sovereign work.

While we carry out the earthly work of nurturing and maintaining our "house," we must remember to consult with the Architect and Builder. Only He knows what really went into the design of your child—your house. We can do all we know how, but as much as we might do in the physical and emotional lives of our children, God is the only one that can work in the spiritual. God wants us to build our families—our "house"—with His wisdom and His ways. He wants to enlighten the eyes of our understanding. (See Ephesians 1:18.)

Proverbs 24:3,4 says, *"By wisdom a house is built, and through understanding it is established; through knowledge its rooms are filled with rare and beautiful treasures."* We find wisdom in God's Word to us. Applying it to our lives brings understanding. Understanding establishes us. When we have searched and discovered revelation or understanding, it means we have taken the truth or wisdom, which may have seemed abstract to us at first, and made it concrete in our hearts and minds. This makes it something we have experienced and not just read. Understanding fixes us so we are unmovable, stable, set, and prepared for what may come.

For example, John 3:16 is truth—God loved us enough to give His only Son, Jesus. We gain salvation from our sins when God reveals that truth to us and establishes us in it. It lets us say, as Paul did, that truly nothing can or will separate us from God's love (Romans 8:38,39). We know that we have eternal life through Jesus Christ because He revealed that understanding to us and because we have experienced God's love.

Proverbs 24:3,4 says that knowledge will fill the rooms of a house—your child—with rare and beautiful treasures. Rare items are of exceptional quality and occur occasionally; sometimes they are unique—one of a kind. Beautiful things draw our attention; we like to be in the company of beautiful things.

Think about the last time you watched a beautiful sunset. I usually find they don't last long enough. Most ladies are not satisfied with just looking at a beautiful diamond; we want to take it out of the showcase and put it on our finger. My husband and I love artwork. It's hard for me to resist touching the different pieces when at an art museum! When we take our children to watch the fireworks on the fourth of July, we are always sad when they are over. They are so beautiful to us—the bright colors, the different shapes, even the loud booms—we don't want them to end. We love it, and we can't wait until next year to see them again.

In the same way we came to understand God's love for us, we must come to understand His wisdom in training our children. We must search for understanding through study and prayer, and we must let that understanding establish us when God reveals it. It will make us unmovable, set, consistent, and decisive in how we train and nurture our children.

The stewardship God gives us over our children doesn't just require us to gain knowledge and understanding from Him, however. We must also be willing to gain knowledge—to educate ourselves—about our children as blossoming individuals. We need to be open to their likes, dislikes, gifts, and abilities. We must pay attention to their personalities and temperaments. When we take time to educate ourselves about our children and how to train them, we will be able to fill the "rooms" of their "houses" with such beautiful and rare treasures that others will be attracted to them.

Obedience Is Not Optional

Fully obeying God's commands is not an option if we are to train and nurture our children successfully. Our family loves to read Deuteronomy chapter 28. It declares to us the promised blessings of God if we fully obey His commands. It says,

> *If you fully obey the LORD your God and carefully follow all his commands I give you today, the LORD your God will set you high above all the nations on earth. All these blessings will come upon you and accompany you if you obey the LORD your God: You will be blessed in the city and blessed in the country. The fruit of your womb will be blessed, and the crops of your land and the young of your livestock—the calves of your herds and the lambs of your flocks. Your basket and your kneading trough will be blessed. You will be blessed when you come in and blessed when you go out.*
>
> Deuteronomy 28:1-6

This is a wonderful promise for parents! However, we need to keep in mind that this only comes when we *fully obey* God's commands. There are sixty-eight verses in the twenty-eighth chapter of Deuteronomy. Most of the time, we never read past the first fourteen—the promises of blessing. When we get to that fifteenth verse and read, "*However, if you do not obey the LORD your God and do not carefully follow all his commands and decrees I am giving you today, all these curses will come upon you and overtake you,*" we often just skip right over the next *fifty-four* verses. There are fourteen about obedience but *fifty-four* about the consequences of disobedience!

We only want to think about the blessings of our obedience. We don't want to acknowledge the consequences of our disobedience. And yet in the same way our obedience brings blessing and favor to the fruit of our womb, our disobedience can nullify the blessing and favor. The Scripture says we will build a house and never enjoy the luxuries of it. We will plant a vineyard and not even begin to enjoy its fruit. Even if we have olive trees, we will never be able to prosper from the oil of their fruit because it will drop before we can harvest it. And the worst for parents—Deuteronomy 28:32 says, *"Your sons and daughters will be given to another nation, and you will wear out your eyes watching for them day after day, powerless to lift a hand."*

Most of us don't plant vineyards, and few of us have sheep to lose to our enemies—it's all figurative anyway—but we have children. God is saying that your disobedience will sell your children off as slaves of this world, away from the Kingdom of God! We will watch them fall away, but there won't be anything we can do if we continue in disobedience; our actions will cost us, and they will cost our children.

Using my previous analogy of the olive trees, planting olive shoots will not produce the oil of anointing in our lives or the lives of those around us if we do not tend them. The anointing will always be just out of reach. Deuteronomy 28 could include a passage that says, "You'll never harvest a drop of oil from your olive orchards; it will fall to the ground before you can try to harvest it."

Obedience is not optional. The consequences to you and your children are just too great.

Perhaps one of the most famous and quoted

❧

Obedience is not optional.

Scriptures about obedience is the story recounted in 1 Samuel chapter 15. God told King Saul through the prophet Samuel to attack the Amalekites and totally destroy them and everything that belonged to them—all the people, all their belongings, and even all their animals! *Everything!*

However, despite God's implicit instructions, Saul does not *fully obey*. He decides to spare Agag, the king of the Amalekites, and to bring back some of the sheep and cattle, the best of which he was going to sacrifice to God.

We can debate his motives all we want. Was his motive noble? Was he trying to do something he thought would please God? Maybe, I'm not sure. I suspect Saul's ego wanted a small victory trophy in King Agag and the sheep and cattle were his idea of compensation for his army's time and energy. Normally they got to keep the spoils of their battles. I also suspect the sacrifice was a diversionary tactic, an attempt to distract God from his disobedience.

However, Saul's motives are irrelevant; the only thing that mattered to God was whether or not he obeyed—fully. And Saul did not. Samuel asks him, *"Why haven't you obeyed the Lord? Why did you rush for the plunder and do exactly what the Lord said not to do?"* in 1 Samuel 15:19 (NLT). Even at this point, Saul argues that he did obey, saying,

> *'But I did obey the LORD,' Saul said. 'I went on the mission the LORD assigned me. I completely destroyed the Amalekites and brought back Agag their king. The soldiers took sheep and cattle from the plunder, the best of what was devoted to God, in order to sacrifice them to the LORD your God at Gilgal.'*

This leads to one of my favorite verses on obedience. In 1 Samuel 15:22,23, Samuel says to Saul,

> *But Samuel replied: 'Does the LORD delight in burnt offerings and sacrifices as much as in obeying the voice of the LORD?* **To obey is better than sacrifice**, *and to heed is better than the fat of rams. For rebellion is like the sin of divination, and arrogance like the evil of idolatry. Because you have rejected the word of the LORD, he has rejected you as king'* (Emphasis added).

Do you remember Psalm 127:4 (NLT), which we looked at earlier? It said, *"Children born to a young man are like sharp arrows in a warrior's hands"*. In Saul's day, men would sometimes throw arrows on the ground in an attempt to find answers to their questions. It was one of their forms of sorcery, witchcraft, or divination. It was man's way of trying to predict outcomes and the future. Rebellion and disobeying God is just like throwing your arrows on the ground, and then instead of being in your quiver, they will be lost to you.

When rebellion is in our heart, we take matters into our own hands and in arrogance attempt to predict our future. We begin to believe our ways are higher than God's ways. Saul's rebellion challenged God's commands. In his arrogance, he thought that because he was doing something that would typically please God, He would ignore his disobedience.

God does not ignore your disobedience—no matter your motives—and it is never acceptable, even when we try to disguise it with noble purposes. Obedience is better than trying to make up for disobedience!

Bringing your children up in this world isn't easy. We're constantly tempted to replace the Word of God with the latest theory on child rearing we saw on a talk show. Often it will seem as though your obedience might cost you something you think you deserve *and you may be tempted to sacrifice as Saul did,* but the rewards for obedience far outweigh whatever you think you might not get! And the consequences of disobedience are not worth it in the end!

Often the rewards we receive for raising our children in a godly manner are not immediate, but we *will* see the fruit of our obedience. Obedience *will* give you all the promised blessings in Deuteronomy 28, and it is our willingness to obey no matter the cost that will keep us eating the best of the land (Isaiah 1:19).

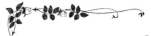 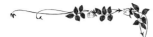

Chapter Three

Parenting: Godly Leadership

As stewards, parents have a mandate from God to teach their children His laws and ways—and to obey Him (Deuteronomy 6:6,7). Moses makes his farewell address to the Children of Israel in Deuteronomy as they wait to cross the Jordan into the land of Canaan. He reminds them to follow the decrees and laws God directed him to teach them. He commands them to love the Lord and to pass down His instructions to their children, and then he proceeds to tell them about the blessings they can expect in the Promised Land.

Deuteronomy 6:6,7 says, *"These commandments that I give you today are to be upon your hearts. Impress them on your children. Talk about them when you sit at home and when you walk along the road, when you lie down and when you get up."* He tells them that first the commands he passed down to them from God needed to be in their hearts, and then he tells them to pass these commands to the hearts of the next generation.

Moses tells them to impart the Lord's ways to their children in every circumstance during any given activity—in other words, all the time. He was saying don't just expect them to learn God's ways in Sunday school; instead, teach your children when you're around the dinner table and when you're driving them to school or to soccer practice or to their ballet recital. When you get up in the morning, let the first thing your children hear you speak be a word of truth; and when you go to bed at night, let the last thing your children hear you speak be a word of truth.

Think of God's law as being tied as symbols on your hands, so that everything you set your hand to do will remind you that you are a leader. Renew your mind with the Word of God so that your attitudes and beliefs will be aligned with the attitudes of God. Let even the entrances of your home remind you, your children, and all others of the standards of your home. Guard the gates of your house from your enemies with the law of God.

One of the strongest examples of godly leadership and parenting in the Bible is that of Abraham and his relationship with Isaac. Remember the circumstances of the story when Abraham nearly sacrificed his son of promise to God out of obedience to God's command.

There they both are on the mountain ready to sacrifice. Isaac was wondering what's up, since they didn't bring a sacrificial lamb with them. When he brought this rather important point to his father's attention earlier, Abraham told him not to worry about it and that God would provide. Isaac didn't bring it up again; he just continued carrying the wood and following his father. Notice he doesn't throw the wood down and scream, "What do you mean 'God will take care of that?' I'm not lugging this wood all the way up the side of this mountain only to have to turn around and come back down because you didn't bring a sacrifice!"

Abraham led, and Isaac followed, and he no doubt easily put two and two together when his father began to tie his hands and feet together. And at this time, Abraham was old and Isaac was probably no longer a little boy—he could have resisted. However, the relationship between Abraham and Isaac had trust as one of its foundation stones. Isaac trusted Abraham; he had no reason not to trust his father.

And Abraham trusted God. He had no reason not to trust Him. Abraham had communicated his covenant and subsequent trust in God in such a way that even when faced with death, Isaac was willing to follow Abraham's lead.

As godly leaders and stewards of God's blessing, everything we are, say, and do represents God and His character to our children. God does not ask us to sacrifice our children on an altar as He did Abraham; Jesus took care of that for us. Abraham's action was a representation of God's heart toward us. Abraham didn't have to sacrifice his son of promise; God sacrificed His Son of promise instead! His Son, Jesus, willingly went to the cross.

Isaac trusted Abraham; Abraham trusted God.

What examples of leadership and obedience! God told Abraham to sacrifice Isaac, and he was going to do it! And Isaac was going to obey and let him. God sacrificed His only Son, and Jesus willingly went to the cross!

God doesn't expect us to be either leaders or followers on our own; we have the Holy Spirit to help us. God doesn't even expect perfection out of us; He knows we're going to mess up and fail. However, even our failure, when we handle it God's way, is an opportunity for us to demonstrate God's love, grace, kindness, forgiveness, and mercy to us so we can model it for our children.

Good leadership incorporates these three principles:

- **Guidance**—Instruction and Training

- **Guardianship**—Protection

- **Government**—Correction and Discipline

A leader should always give clear and concise directions. He should ensure that those following him are taught and trained for the task they are being assigned. The leader should always be there in case of attack, and he should guarantee to the best of his ability their safety while they are carrying out their assigned task. One of the ways he provides protection is through correction and discipline. If those following him deviate from the instruction and training, the leader should guide them back to the correct path with appropriate consequences. He should establish clear and fair guidelines.

Since we, as parents, are leaders to our children, these principles can and should be applied to our parenting styles. Our children must know without a doubt we will defend them, be on their side, and protect them to the best of our ability from all physical, emotional, and spiritual danger. We must communicate clear, concise, and age-appropriate instructions at every stage in our children's development. By establishing fair guidelines (call them rules if you want to) we protect our children—as well as teach them that there are rewards for obedience and consequences for every disobedience.

One of the best ways you can govern your children is to give them a vision for which they can reach. Proverbs 29:17,18 says, *"Discipline your son, and he will give you peace; he will bring delight to your soul. Where there is no revelation, the people cast off restraint; but blessed is he who keeps the law."* Habakkuk 2:2 says, *"Then the LORD replied: 'Write down the revelation and make it plain on tablets so that a herald may run with it.'"*

Some years ago my husband and I decided to ask God what His purpose was for our family. We wanted to know what we were supposed to be representing to those around us. We asked ourselves, "What are the bottom-line principles we want to instill in the hearts of our children?"

A vision gives direction and purpose, and we decided that the first part of discipline for us and for our children was to establish a basic vision for our family.

A vision gives you direction, which in turn gives you something on which to base your discipline—a standard. When you don't have direction, you open the door to anarchy. Direction and discipline help your children learn to exercise self-control.

From these assumptions, we wrote the following:

Our Family Vision

It is the vision of our family to live life to the fullest by the power of the Holy Spirit; to be agents of God's Kingdom, bringing restoration through our collective lives; and to be committed to bringing out the best in each other through instruction, encouragement, prayer, and speaking the truth in love. We will not only minister God's redemptive love to each other but to all those we come in contact with. Remembering always we are a family (city) set on a hill, we will endeavor to live lives worthy of our calling. We walk by faith not by sight and choose to believe the report of the Lord!

By writing down your family's vision, you give each family member something concrete to hold on to. Your vision will give direction to your family and meaning to your discipline; it will also give your family members goals and something for which to strive.

Your family vision doesn't have to be poetic, wordy, or in King James English. Joshua's family vision was simple and straight to the point: *"As for me and my house, we will serve the Lord"* (Joshua 24:15b). Joshua made it clear that idolatry wasn't acceptable in his household.

Your family vision might only be a list of Scriptures that reflect God's desires for your family. Here are some examples of some Scriptures that would make excellent components for your family vision, but there are countless numbers of excellent verses from which you can choose.

- *"Let love and faithfulness never leave you; bind them around your neck, write them on the tablet of your heart.*
  Proverbs 3:3
- *"This is my command: Love each other."*
  John 15:17
- *"But I tell you: Love your enemies and pray for those who persecute you."*
  Matthew 5:44
- *"Give thanks to the Lord, for he is good."*
  Psalm 136:1
- *"Enter his gates with thanksgiving and his courts with praise; give thanks to him and praise his name."*
  Psalm 100:4
- *"If one falls down, his friend can help him up. But pity the man who falls and has no one to help him up."*
  Ecclesiastes 4:10
- *"Do not let any unwholesome talk come out of your mouths, but only what is helpful for building others up according to their needs."*
  Ephesians 4:29

There are many books available that list Scriptures under specific headings and topics in most Christian bookstores; these are ideal resources for finding the verses that you might like to use in your family vision.

Also, don't feel as though you must sit down *right now* and write out the perfect vision statement for your family. You may want to build it gradually by just jotting down Scriptures you come across in your daily study of the Word of God.

Once you've written your vision, put it someplace where it is highly visible. You might want to make several copies and place them in key locations throughout your house so all those who see and read it may run with it.

Be an Example

Remember, your children will follow your lead—whether you want them to or not. The real issue then is being a godly leader. We partially discussed this earlier, but I'd like to reiterate that the greatest teaching tool you have is not your ability to exercise authority over your children; it's the example you set for them.

The Apostle Paul knew the importance of being a godly example to those under his authority. In 1 Corinthians Paul wrote to a church that was coming out of paganism. The Corinthian Christians were dealing with changing their lifestyle and learning to live a godly and holy lifestyle.

Paul begins his letter by stating that he is an apostle of Jesus Christ, establishing his authority. In the same manner, your children must understand your authority over them; but remember, they will follow your example, not your authority. Paul understood this, and in chapter 11, he says that the Corinthians should follow him as he follows Christ. He established his authority, set their guidelines, and then told them to follow his godly example.

> *Your children will follow your lead—whether you want them to or not.*

Paul even likens himself to a parent rather than simply an authority figure. He addressed their problems not only as a guardian but a father to his sons and daughters (1 Corinthians 4:14-17). In essence, he said, "I brought you into the Kingdom of God. I'm not only here to give counsel and guidelines, I love you. I am your spiritual father, and I'm not going anywhere. You can trust what I say, and I have your best interest at the center of my heart."

As godly leaders to our children, we cannot be guardians without also being fathers and mothers. We cannot nurture and train our children with legalistic ideas and hearts; your guardianship must flow from your love for them, just as Christ's flows from His love for us.

Paul's letter to the Corinthians is not the only time he likens his leadership to that of a parent. He addressed similar issues in 2 Thessalonians. There were some people in the Thessalonian church who were not following Paul's example. He told the church to remove themselves from these men and to follow after the example he set before them. He reminded the church that he too was living the teachings he brought them. Paul backed up his spoken words with actions; he lived what he preached.

The first step in becoming a godly leader to your children is to understand how important your example is to them. I've heard parents say to their children, "You just do what I say, not what I do." It's an understatement to say this doesn't work! Sometimes adults have privileges that children do not, and we are not always able to satisfactorily explain these privileges to our children. But if you are continually mandating a certain standard for your children that you are not also adhering to, you will build resentment in them.

First Peter 5:1-3 describes the leadership strategy for elders in the Church, but it is the same for parents:

> *To the elders among you, I appeal as a fellow elder, a witness of Christ's sufferings and one who also will share in the glory to be revealed: be shepherds of God's flock that is*

under your care, serving as overseers—not because you must, but because you are willing, as God wants you to be; not greedy for money, but eager to serve; not lording it over those entrusted to you, but being examples to the flock.

We are to lead them by example. If you want your children to learn to be submissive, then you must submit to the authority God has placed in your life. Authority comes from submission, and God has established a chain of command by which you get your authority over your children. But you must lead them by your actions as well as your words.

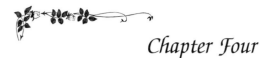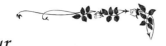

Chapter Four

Learning to Love

When I married my husband, I believed I really loved him. And I did love him; but the longer we are together, the more we *learn* how to love each other. We soon realized that love was not really all about the butterflies and warm fuzzies. Learning to love is a process. We must learn how to love each other, and we must learn how to love our children.

Titus 2:4 (NLT) says that *"older women must* **train** *the younger women to* **love** *their* **husbands** *and their* **children"** (Emphasis added). Paul was speaking about women teaching younger women in particular, but the principle applies to everyone. If we already knew how to love our spouses and our children, why would Paul give special instructions in this area? Evidently, the kind of love that Paul knows we need isn't automatic; we have to learn it.

Whatever the circumstances that made Paul decide to give special instructions, today we have many people in our society who have handicaps in the love department. Many of us have been raised in less than ideal home environments. Countless people arrive at adulthood without a foundation of love and support in their lives.

And then we meet Jesus, and He causes us to experience love such as we have never known. His love is the greatest example we have, and our understanding of true love comes only when we begin to understand His love.

I believe one of the most comprehensive Scriptures on love is in 1 John 4:7-19. Let's take a look at it and then the specific elements within it.

> *Dear friends, let us love one another, for love comes from God. Everyone who loves has been born of God and knows God. Whoever does not love does not know God, because God is love. This is how God showed his love among us: He sent his one and only Son into the world that we might live through him. This is love: not that we loved God, but that he loved us and sent his Son as an atoning sacrifice for our sins. Dear friends, since God so loved us, we also ought to love one another. No one has ever seen God; but if we love one another, God lives in us and his love is made complete in us. We know that we live in him and he in us, because he has given us of his Spirit. And we have seen and testify that the Father has sent his Son to be the Savior of the world. If anyone acknowledges that Jesus is the Son of God, God lives in him and he in God. And so we know and rely on the love God has for us. God is love. Whoever lives in love lives in God, and God in him. In this way, love is made complete among us so that we will have confidence on the day of judgment, because in this world we are like him. There is no fear in love. But perfect love drives out fear, because fear has to do with punishment. The one who fears is not made perfect in love. We love because he first loved us.*

There are four things in this passage I want us to look at in greater depth. They will give a good picture of how God loves and therefore how we should love.

◆ **He has given us His Holy Spirit.**

Galatians 6:22 tells us about the fruit of the Spirit. Love is part of that fruit, and our lives should demonstrate it. Love is evidence that the Holy Spirit is working in and through you. The Holy Spirit was sent to bring comfort, guidance, and to speak the will of the Father to us. When we choose to listen and obey the voice of the Spirit, *He* will tell us how to love—even when we aren't sure how.

When faced with disciplining your children, He will speak to your heart how best to go about it. He will show how to best encourage your children and how to demonstrate your affection toward them. Our Father God knew we would need help—all we must do is listen and obey Him. Let the Holy Spirit be your partner; God doesn't expect you to be able to do it in your own strength. (See also John 16:7, 13-15, Acts 1:8, Acts 2:1-4.)

◆ **God's love is reliable.**

We have heard that God loves us so many times, many Christians never really doubt His love toward them. We may feel we don't deserve it, but the Bible tells that nothing can separate it from us (Romans 8:35–39). This is how we are to love our children—they must know that nothing can separate

Children need the stability your love provides.

them from our love for them, and that we will always be there to love and encourage them. Children need the stability your love provides. They must know that whether they succeed or fail, your love is there to cheer them on or to break their fall.

One way we assure our children of our love is through verbal expressions of love. You can never say "I love you" enough! We reaffirm our love for them when we verbalize our feelings toward them. Verbalize your love to them directly and to others as well—especially within their hearing. My husband and I started a habit each night with our children early in their lives. Every night as we put them to bed, the last thing we would say to them was, "Who loves you more than anyone in the whole, wide world?" to which they would respond, "Mommy and Daddy!" We would then ask them, "Who loves you most of all?" Their response was, "Jesus!" As of the writing of this book, they would still answer those questions the same way. Your children will remember your love long after they move out to start their own homes.

◆ **God's love produces confidence.**

I hear a lot of talk these days about how important building self-esteem and confidence is; kids seem to often lack both. Helping your child develop these two attributes is especially important, and the foundation for a child's confidence and self-assuredness is your godly love. God's love in us makes us more confident as we walk by faith and experience His plan for our lives, and when we provide our children with reliable love they will begin to feel positively about themselves and become confident.

A mature Christian knows that God is there for him and that failing doesn't mean being a failure. So too, when your children know they are unconditionally loved, they will not be afraid to try, even if they fail. The more I experience God's love, the more confidently I am able to walk out His plan for my life. When we provide our children with the same kind of love, they will begin to feel positively about themselves and walk more confidently into their future.

Take a moment and reread 1 John 4:17 from earlier in the chapter. It says that as our love grows more perfect (more Christlike), we can have confidence on the day of judgment because we rely on God's love. If you've taught your children the same thing, when their many days of judgment come, they will be able to be confident and face the consequences and rewards of their behavior. The foundation of unconditional and reliable love you lay in their lives produces your children's self-esteem and confidence.

◆ **There is no fear in love.**

Fear is the opposite of faith. The two cannot coexist; fear robs you of your ability to function as God intends. You will find fear at the root of many issues with which people struggle. Children without a foundation of love from God and their parents are usually fearful. I'm not talking about kids who are timid or bashful; I'm talking about children who suffer from a spirit of fear. Gregarious people can be full of fear—often, their outgoing exterior masks their insecurities. Children often disguise their fear with humor or aggressive behavior.

A spirit of fear ultimately immobilizes people and results in an ineffective and unproductive life. It causes people to live in lack in spirit, soul, and body. However, as 1 John 4:18 says, the kind of love God wants us to cultivate drives fear out! When godly love drives out fear, it replaces it with faith.

God never intended for us to have a spirit of fear. He intends for us to walk in one of power, love, and a strong mind (2 Timothy 1:7). Just as faith and fear cannot abide in the same house, so love and fear cannot! Your faith—and your children's—works through love (Galatians 5:6), because love drives the fear out!

God's Definition of Love

We've looked at a scriptural example of how God loves in 1 John 4; now let's look at His definition of love. I find the greatest written definition of love in 1 Corinthians 13. Here is a portion of that chapter:

> *Love is patient, love is kind. It does not envy, it does not boast, it is not proud. It is not rude, it is not self-seeking, it is not easily angered, it keeps no record of wrongs. Love does not delight in evil but rejoices with the truth. It always protects, always trusts, always hopes, always perseveres.*
>
> 1 Corinthians 13:4-7

♦ **Love is patient.**

The word *patient* means, "bearing misfortune, provocation, annoyance, delay, hardship, pain, etc. with fortitude and calm and without anger, complaint or the like" (Webster's Encyclopedic Unabridged Dictionary). That can seem like a pretty tall order. Children, just because they are children, have a way of provoking, annoying, delaying, and inflicting hardship—and occasionally pain—on their parents.

Parents' lives are filled with opportunities to lose their patience. Most parents can attest to the misfortune of having planned a big evening out only to suddenly discover their daughter, Susie, develops a fever of 102 and an earache—there goes the big night.

Your child shouts, "I want Grandma to put my shoes on!" to which you calmly reply, "Sweetheart, Grandma can't right now; she's busy." You get the reply, "*I want GRANDMA!*" and suddenly, you're provoked.

You want to make a quick run to the store for milk before dinner, and your son wants to come. Junior wants to tie his own shoes, but of course it takes him ten minutes for each shoe. Your offer to help only brings greater resolve to him doing it *all by himself.* And just like that, you're annoyed.

I have a tendency to run late to begin with, and just about the time I smile at the thought of being on time, one of my kids throws up, spills a drink, or breaks something, guaranteeing my tardiness once again—a recipe for delay.

Just ask the mother who's had her infant rip an earring out of her pierced ear or the father who, while teaching his son to play baseball, gets hit in the shin (or someplace worse) with the bat; these parents will tell you all about pain.

I won't even attempt to cover the provocation, annoyances, delays, hardships, and pain that most teenagers inflict on their parents. And of course there is the heart pain parents often feel when their children make wrong choices or disappoint them.

Yet because we love them, we must be patient. Love really is patient—or at least it must be working toward being patient. Learning to be patient is a process, and the beginning of the process is knowing and understanding that true love shows patience.

Children are children, and they are going to go through many necessary—and frustrating—stages of growth and development. They are going to make mistakes. Take time to research the stages of growth and development your children are going to go through so they don't take you by surprise. Knowing what is normal and appropriate behavior and attitudes for your child's stage is half the battle of learning to be patient.

For example, it is unrealistic to expect your tremendous two-year-old to sit still and be quiet for any length of time without some form—more accurately forms—of entertainment. Knowing this ahead of time enables you to prepare for and thus avoid being provoked and annoyed at his behavior in a restaurant.

We can patiently guide our children through the stages of childhood. You just have to be patient. And don't rush it; they'll only be this age once, and then it will be gone.

♦ **Love is not self-seeking.**

Just the cold hard facts here—you are periodically going to have to give up something of yourself for the sake of the children. True love understands that when children enter the scene, life changes. Sleep schedules become more important than ever, and you can't always do the things you want to when you want to do them. You just have to adjust, love them, and be patient. You might as well relax—you're most likely going to be practicing your patience for the rest of their lives.

Many times have I heard expecting parents declare, "Life is not going to change for us. We're just going to take our precious bundle of joy with us wherever we go." Veteran parents laugh heartily at that one. They know the work involved in taking the "precious bundle of joy" with them everywhere they go. Stacks of diapers, bottles, pacifiers, blankets, five changes of clothes, portable cribs, strollers, backpack carriers—the list goes on and on.

You may remember when it was easy to go to the all-day-long church softball tournament? Now your youngest precious one won't take her nap and is screaming her head off and your toddler, Sammy, keeps trying to eat the rocks, trash and other treasures he finds on the ground. Parents of elementary-age children and teenagers know well the amount of time and energy they dedicate first to their children's spiritual training—to keep them focused and on track—and second to their daily schedules. I am convinced adolescents believe their parents' true purpose in life is to transport them from one friend's house to another and from activity to activity.

Am I saying you will never have fun again or that life as you know it completely disappears after kids? No—not really. However, what I am saying is that true godly love is sacrificial (John 15:13). Real love and self-indulgence are usually mutually exclusive; they can't coexist any more than fear and faith can.

Love means that you begin taking others' needs into consideration before your own—whether it's love for your children or your spouse; that's God's way. Jesus said,

> *'Love the Lord your God with all your heart and with all your soul and with all your mind.' This is the first and greatest commandment. And the second is like it: 'Love your neighbor as yourself.' All the Law and the Prophets hang on these two commandments.*
>
> Matthew 22:37-40

♦ **Love is not easily angered.**

Opportunities to get angry present themselves to us every day, and children seem to be catalysts for stirring up anger. First, it is not wrong to experience the feeling of anger. It is wrong when we respond inappropriately to our feeling, and we never want to be *easily* angered. The Bible is full of instruction about anger. Psalm 4:4 (NLT) says, *"Don't sin by letting anger gain control over you."* The New King James Version puts that verse as, *"Be angry, and do not sin."* You can be angry without sinning; it's what you do with your anger that's important—if you're angry, don't let it make you sin.

Recall our Scripture from 1 Corinthians chapter 13. The King James Version reads that love *"is not easily provoked"* (1 Corinthians 13:5). Let's focus on the word *easily*. The word *easily* refers to something happening without much effort; it comes naturally to you. The more you practice something, the easier it becomes for you to do it. Anger is not an emotion you should be practicing. It should not be easy for someone to stir up anger in you.

Modern psychology rightly attests that no one can *make* you do, feel, or be *anything*. No one can *make* you angry. You choose when, where, and to what degree you exercise your emotions. People can make it *easy* for you to become angry, but they can't make you. Not even your children can *make* you angry.

This is not to say that you won't—and shouldn't— ever be angry. It's appropriate to respond with anger to certain circumstances; Jesus demonstrates this for us in His response to the complete disrespect and dishonesty He found in the temple court (John 2:13-17). He was angry and showed it quite forcefully. Yet in the story of His life here on earth, this is the only time we see anger like this from Jesus. Obviously, He was not easily angered.

Don't let your children anger you. Practice not get-ting angry so that staying calm is easy instead of it being easy to get angry. Save your anger for when it really matters. Save it for those moments when it will effectively communicate your message and serve a purpose. Jesus' anger served a purpose and got His message across— what they were doing was

Jesus was not easily angered.

unacceptable. And when He was done driving sin from the Temple, He turned His attention to healing the blind and the lame.

Properly used and channeled anger can be a good thing, despite its stigma as a negative emotion. We must simply exercise self-control and not sin when we are angry. Don't get angry over spilled milk.

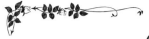 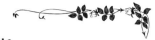

Chapter Five

Praying for Your Children

Prayer, very simply, is talking to and listening to God. It is communication between God and His children. Edwin Keith in *A Man's Work Is Never Done* said prayer is exhaling the spirit of man and inhaling the Spirit of God. I like that. It means there is an *exchange* happening. As I talk with my Father God, little by little the frailties of my humanity are exchanged for the greatness and strengths of His power. We must take time to talk with God regularly to keep the exchange ongoing and strong in our lives. The strength of the exchange is in our spirit touching and being refreshed by touching the Spirit of God.

The responsibility of parenting can seem overwhelming at times. If we rely on our abilities and strength, they will eventually become taxed and fall short. Philippians 4:4-7 says,

> *Rejoice in the Lord always. I will say it again: Rejoice! Let your gentleness be evident to all. The Lord is near. Do not be anxious about anything, but in everything, by prayer and petition, with thanksgiving, present your requests to God. And the peace of God, which transcends all understanding, will guard your hearts and your minds in Christ Jesus.*

Present your requests—all of them, parenting included—to God. God says not to become anxious or begin to worry but to make our request known to Him. His peace, which we can't begin to understand or describe, will guard us. He promises He is always near, willing, and able to answer and provide for our needs. Let me say right from the beginning of this chapter, if you haven't prayed specifically for yourself and your responsibilities as a parent, begin to do so now. God will hear and answer your prayers!

Here are just a few reasons to pray that I find personally meaningful.

- **Pray for wisdom and revelation** to come to you concerning the training of your children. To train our children according to the Word of God, we must know it and have God reveal it.
- **Pray for strength and courage** to stand your ground. Opportunities to back down from the Word of truth and household standards present themselves constantly. Pray God will give you strength in your soul (emotions, will, decision making) to resist the temptation. Remember, obedience is not optional, but He is with you, and through Him you can do all things.
- **Pray that the fruit of the Spirit will rule in your spirit.** (See Galatians 5:22,23.)
- **Pray that God uses you to encourage yourself and others**. Be purposefully positive and not negative, and ask that He make you a "half full" rather than a "half empty" kind of person.
- **Pray that God will stir the gift of faith in you.** Faith works through love, and without faith, it is impossible to please God (Hebrews 11:6).
- **Pray that God will make you an overcomer** (John 16:33; 1 John 5:4,5).

Three Parts of Prayer

1) Praise & Worship

Begin your prayer time with sincere praise and worship. Let it come from deep within you. There is a song on the inside of you God wants to hear! Worship and praise Him because of who He is to you personally. Talk to Him, sing to Him, wait on Him to come and speak to you. Listen carefully to hear His voice as He speaks to you.

2) Petition

Our God will supply our needs according to *His* riches, not ours. When you have needs, whether material or spiritual, He is faithful to hear and answer when we pray according to His will. Do not hesitate to ask God to meet your personal needs and those of your family.

3) Thanksgiving

Psalm 136:1 tells us to give thanks to the Lord because He is good. David said we should enter His gates with thanksgiving (Psalm 100:4). Philippians 4:6 says that when we ask for God to meet our needs, we must ask with thanksgiving in our hearts. Do not forget to thank God for meeting needs and for just being good to you!

Why Pray?

We see an example of God's presence dwelling with a man in Moses' life. Moses spent a great deal of time communing with God. He knew the power of knowing God intimately. He understood the effect of God's presence in his life so well that at one point he declared that he wouldn't go anywhere unless God's presence went before him. Abraham also spent a great amount of time communing with God. It's no wonder God called him His friend!

When we communicate with God, His presence comes to dwell with us. In God's presence, we find fullness of joy, peace that surpasses our understanding, strength, love, revelation, the fruit of the Spirit, and much more. We find everything we need by knowing Him (2 Peter 1:3).

As you fulfill your role as parent, there will be times when you are uncertain as to how to deal with situations. Jeremiah 33:2,3 tells us our God is the one who created everything and that if we call out to Him, He will answer and show us great and mighty things we do not know. We can ask God to show us what we do not know! There will be times when you won't know what to do and with which no parenting book can help you. But when you don't know what to do, *God* does! So don't stress out; just ask.

We can have confidence that God is willing and able to meet our needs. Jesus taught His disciples how to pray in Luke 11. After teaching them what we refer to as the Lord's Prayer, He further explained that as His children, we have a right to ask when we have need. God wants to meet your needs, and He promises that everyone who asks receives!

Jesus frequently used the analogy of a relationship between father and son. As parents, we can relate to this. When our children ask for something and it is not harmful to them and within our power to give it to them, why would we not grant their request? I doubt that many parents get their children the complete opposite toy they ask for, and in the same vein, God wants to grant our requests. Perhaps you've waited in line for that must-have Christmas toy and after enduring long lines, finally managed to put it under your tree. If so, you probably know firsthand the great joy of watching delight spread across your child's face on Christmas morning as he or she opens the paper and finds their treasure. The squeals of delight, dances of joy, and hugs and kisses make any inconvenience worth it.

We love watching our children take joy in receiving the desires of their heart, and our heavenly Father takes great pleasure in watching us celebrate His blessings as well. But the Kingdom of God works slightly different than the kingdom of this world. God is our provider, but our need alone is not what moves Him to meet the desires of our heart. Our faith moves Him.

Our need alone is not what moves Him to meet the desires of our heart. Our faith moves Him.

When we have needs and exercise our faith in asking for those needs, God moves on our behalf. He wants to!

Praying for Your Children

When you begin to pray for your children, stick to the Word of God. The Word is sure and everlasting. We can fully rely on it and know it will do what it was sent to do (Isaiah 55:11). Jesus said if we abide or live in Him and His Word lives in us, we can ask what we need and He'll do it (John 15:7). Our words may fail, and the words of others may fail us, but God's Word to us will never fail!

If you are praying for specific problems or needs, do not pray the problem; pray for the solution. God knows the situation, and He's Jehovah-Jireh, your provider! Exercise your faith, and confess the Word of Truth over the problem. It is easy for our prayers to become gripe sessions or for our prayers to be no more than another note in the complaint box of our lives. So don't get distracted by the problem; stick to the Word and its promises.

Let me give you an example that might be helpful. Let's say that your son is having difficulty telling the truth. Don't spend all your time telling God about how tired you are of Junior's behavior. God knows how frustrated you are. He knows you feel as though you are at your wit's end and have had it up to here. Instead of belaboring God with your frustration, move on to something constructive. Move on to something that will actually bring change to the situation. I've included the Scripture references for certain portions of the prayer that are directly according to the Word. Here is an example you might use:

> Father, I come to you in Jesus' name, asking you for wisdom and understanding concerning my son's lying. Father, I pray that your righteousness will grow in him and that he will begin to speak only those things that are right and true (Isaiah 33:15). Let him be a man of value who speaks only what is truth (Proverbs 16:13). Help me to teach him the benefits of truth. I ask you to give me wisdom in how to bring correction and discipline to Junior when he needs it. I'm so glad that what concerns me concerns You, and I know You will help me with this situation. Give me an ear to hear what You speak to me, and the courage to obey. Thank You for hearing and answering me!

When you pray, attach mountain-moving faith to your prayers. That kind of faith yields results—mountains in your life will move and be cast into the sea (Mark 11:22-24). Remember, nothing is too difficult for God!

I believe we should ask God for supernatural protection for our children. I believe one of the best ways to do this is by praying according to Psalm 91. It is easy to insert the names of your children or whole family in this particular passage. Let me use my children as an example:

> Meredith and Stephen dwell in the shelter of the Most High and will rest in the shadow of You, Lord, the Almighty. They will say of the Lord, "He is our refuge and our fortress, our God, in whom we trust." Surely, You, Lord, will save Meredith and Stephen from the fowler's snare and from deadly pestilence. You will cover Meredith and Stephen with Your feathers and under Your wings they will find refuge. They will not fear the terror of night, nor the arrow that flies by day….

You can use this same passage to pray for your whole family. It is such a wonderful and complete way to pray for protection using the Word of God!

Proverbs 22:6 (NKJV) says, *"Train up a child in the way he should go, and when he is old he will not depart from it."* God has a way that your children should go. That way is His purpose for their lives. God spoke to Jeremiah (Jeremiah 1:5) and said while he was in his mother's womb that he was appointed to be a prophet to the nations.

Not all of our children may be prophets to the nations, but God has appointed to them their own unique tasks. God has set them apart for a purpose in His Kingdom. God saw past what Jeremiah thought were hindrances (his lack of knowledge and youthfulness) and spoke straight to the destiny locked up inside of him. God reminded Jeremiah that He equips those He appoints for a particular purpose.

As we pray for our children, we must begin to ask God to show us what particular way He has for each of our children to go. God has set your children apart for His own purposes; ask Him what they are. Ask God to begin to reveal your child's purpose.

In some instances, God may show us a definite career or occupation for our children, but more often He will speak about their strengths and abilities. The *way* your child should go has more to do with the *manner* in which he goes than the particular occupation he chooses. When we see strengths or particular abilities in our children, we must know how to promote and encourage those strengths and abilities. Pray that God shows you how to promote and encourage God's purpose in their lives.

One young child I know has a strong compassion for souls. He is always thinking about those who have not accepted Jesus as their Savior. One day as his mother prayed for him, she began to thank God that her son had such a great love for the unsaved. God spoke to her and said, "I placed that great love in his young heart. Be sure he knows what My Word says about salvation. Be sure he knows how to lead someone to Me." Immediately she went about teaching him Scriptures on salvation and making certain he understood the power of what Jesus did on the cross.

He may grow up and walk out the office of an evangelist, or he may be a teacher who has a great gift for evangelism. Or maybe he'll work in the marketplace but be a witness to everyone around him. We don't know at this point, but we do know God will use this great love for the unsaved in some way. His parents are training him in that way—the way of someone with a heart to evangelize.

God is setting your children apart for His purposes, and when you pray and ask Him to reveal His hand in their lives, you can participate by raising them with His goals in mind. You can help impart this sense of purpose into your children. Mostly, though, you want to train your children so that as they grow and mature, they too will seek the purpose of God for their lives.

Many aspects of training your children apply to every child—building their character and helping them develop their own relationship with God and moral compass. However, I believe that you can be an active participant in bringing about God's specific course for your child.

You can be an active participant in bringing about God's specific course for your child.

Ask Him to show you why your child was born and to help you begin to uncover your child's purpose.

It is this kind of understanding that can initiate the purposes of God in the lives of our children, and it comes through direct communication between you and God. We begin by sowing the seeds of understanding, and as they grow and mature, they too will seek out and follow after the purpose of God for their lives.

Here is an example of a prayer similar to what I would pray for my children. Maybe it will help you if you are just beginning to pray for your children. Simply fill in your children's names, and you have something to get you started.

> Father, I come to You in the name of Jesus, praying for Meredith and Stephen. I believe that You are causing them to know You personally and intimately. Thank You Lord that they are learning to hear and respond to Your voice and that Meredith and Stephen are learning to love You with all their hearts, souls, and minds. I pray, Father, that a spirit of love joy and peace will surround them and that

Your presence will go before them, opening doors that no man can shut. I thank You Lord that Your face is turned toward them and Your favor gives them favor with man. I believe that Meredith and Stephen are children of destiny and will fulfill their God-given purpose on the earth. I know You, not man, have ordered their steps and that they delight in Your ways. I thank You that Meredith and Stephen are children of honor and obedience, able and willing to receive correction and instruction. Thank you that they are children of Your Word able to rightly divide the Word of Truth. I pray that they will be as bold as lions and gentle as lambs. I believe that Meredith and Stephen will speak the Word of the Lord in love, with all the boldness, courage, strength, and authority that You have given them. I pray that Meredith and Stephen will be well-learned children and live up to their full potential. The law of kindness is on their tongues and they are wellsprings of life to everyone with whom they come into contact. I thank You, Lord, that Meredith and Stephen do not walk after the counsel of the ungodly, or stand in the way of sinners, or sit in the seat of mockers, but delight in You and that You are causing everything to which they set their hands to prosper and be fruitful. Thank you they are fruitful vines. I ask You, Lord, to set Your angels around Meredith and Stephen to guard them in all their ways. We know that because we have made You our dwelling place, You will not allow snares or deadly pestilence to prosper against our family. Your faithfulness will be their shield, and we will not fear. You love them, Father, and I believe You will rescue

Meredith and Stephen and protect them. We will acknowledge that You are our salvation and give You all honor and praise. I thank You for hearing and answering my prayers, and for delivering and honoring this family. Thank you that long life and salvation will be in this house because we choose to put You first and will continue to declare that You are the Lord of our lives as individuals and as a family.

You probably should also pray for other areas of concern such as:

- That they will make good choices regarding their friends
- That they will have healthy emotions
- That they will stay pure and holy
- That they will have godly discernment and wisdom
- That they would be filled with the Holy Spirit and receive their prayer language
- That God will be with them regarding their specific problems
- That He would break any generational curses
- That they would be free from fear
- That they would avoid addictions
- That they develop self-control
- That they would grow in their faith

Especially if you are just beginning to pray for your children, it is good to start with a basic outline. But listen to the leading of the Holy Spirit. He will lead you to pray for specific things—sometimes things for which you would not normally know to pray—for your children. Also, it is good to spend time praying in the Spirit for your children.

Praying With Your Children

It is not only important that you pray *for* your children; it's important that you pray *with* your children. When we pray with our children, it will develop a deeper more intimate relationship—one of a spiritual nature. Something supernatural happens when you and your child sit down together to worship and talk with God!

As you pray together, your children will begin to see and understand the anointing of God in your life—

ᔧᕯᔦ

It's important that you pray with your children.

you'll demonstrate your relationship with God. When they discern the anointing in your life, God will begin to transfer it to them, also. They'll begin to participate in it. This transferred anointing will become tangible to your children as you pray with them.

We see this principle in the life of Abraham. God told Abraham that He would bless those who blessed him and curse those who cursed him (Genesis 12:3). Those who recognized the blessing of God on Abraham's life and connected themselves with that blessing became blessed themselves! Abraham is the one to whom the Word of God came and the one with whom God made the covenant of promise.

For example, Abraham's nephew Lot connected himself with Abraham, and the blessing that God spoke over Abraham's life carried over into the lives of Lot and his family. Even when Abraham made a mistake in Egypt, Lot stuck with him and did not leave. Genesis 13:5 says that Lot *"who was moving about with Abraham, also had flocks and herds and tents."* And Lot didn't have anything before he hooked up with Abraham. As he followed

Abraham, he also prospered—being around Abraham yielded blessings for Lot!

Abraham and Lot both prospered to the point that there was not room for them to dwell in close proximity, and quarreling broke out between their herdsmen. Abraham tells Lot, "I don't want quarreling between you and me, so maybe we should separate." Now Lot had a choice here. He could fix the problem by stopping the quarreling, working out the troubles and stay connected to Abraham and the blessing; or he could leave. He chose the latter and left.

Abraham gave him the choice between two places: one looks blessed and prosperous to the natural eye (plain of Jordan) and the other (Canaan) does not. Lot chose the plain of Jordan, the place that appears blessed to him. Unfortunately, there is a little place called Sodom and another little place called Gomorrah there.

Lot lost his freedom and his possessions when Sodom and Gomorrah fall in war, and Abraham rescued Lot and recovered his goods. This restored Lot to the place of blessing because of what Abraham did.

The next time we read about Lot again, he was disconnected from Abraham once more. This time, he was in a worse position than before. He was in Sodom, a cursed place, attempting to be blessed. God was ready to destroy Sodom and Gomorrah, and Lot too, but Abraham interceded for him. Abraham, the man with the anointing, again rescued him. But this time, Lot loses everything—including his wife, who turns back in longing for the cursed, sinful city and turns into a pillar of salt. Lot and his two daughters end up living in a cave in the mountains. Some very unseemly things go on, and his daughters become pregnant by him. And the Moabites and Ammonites, which become enemies to Abraham's descendents, the Children of Israel, are the result of that unholy union.

Now here is the connection: had Lot continued to recognize and acknowledge the anointing (blessing) of God on Abraham's life, he would have continued in the same anointing. When we pray with our children, we give them access to the anointing of God in *our* lives. As they discern that anointing and acknowledge it in our lives, it can transfer to their lives.

In 2 Timothy 1:5 Paul reminds Timothy where his sincere faith began. It began in his grandmother, Lois. Her daughter Eunice received this faith also, and she passed it on in turn to Timothy. God will pass on the good things in your family—your faith and anointing—to your children when we take time to reveal His work in us. One of the greatest opportunities for this is in our prayer time with them. They will see your sincere love and intimacy with God, up close and personal.

Praying together creates family unity; simply living in the same house is not the same as living together as a family unit. David writes about how wonderful living in unity is in Psalm 133 (NKJV), describing it in poetic terms. He writes,

> *Behold, how good and how pleasant it is for brethren to dwell together in unity! It is like the precious oil upon the head, running down on the beard, the beard of Aaron, running down on the edge of his garments. It is like the dew of Hermon, descending upon the mountains of Zion; for there the Lord commanded the blessing—life forevermore.*

Unity means as one; it has to do with joining more than one thing together in such a way that those separate things now function as one.

For example, our natural bodies consist of many separate body systems, organs—all the way down to tissues and cells. Cells of uniform function form tissues; tissues working together are organs; organs work together as systems; and finally the various systems working in unity are one fully-functioning body.

When we live together in unity (as one), the anointing that is poured out upon the head of the family flows downward. The anointing doesn't flow over those who are near; it flows to those who are under the head and connected to it.

You as a parent are a spiritual leader for your family—you are the head. Notice in the Psalm that the oil starts at the top of the head and flows down to the beard and collar. God's anointing starts with you, but it flows down your family, covering them each in turn when they are in unity and under your leadership and authority.

The disciples asked Jesus how to pray, and from that, we have the Lord's Prayer. Praying with your children not only provides them an example, it will teach them *how* to pray. They will learn from listening to you talk to God.

God's anointing starts with you, but it flows down your family.

It's important to pray in normal language when you're praying with your kids. In fact, use it as a way of getting away from praying as though you're in the sixteenth century. There is nothing more holy about praying in King James English; it doesn't get God's attention more than speaking the way you would to anyone else. Talk to God in the same manner you would talk to your other family members. Keep in mind that your children are learning from your example, and they won't be able to talk King James. We want them to understand that while Father God is to be revered, He is easily and completely accessible to them!

Praying with your children enables them to rejoice with you over answered prayers. This will build their faith! As you pray together as a family, take time to pray for the needs of others as well as the needs of your immediate family. Encourage your children to approach God with their own needs in the same way we discussed earlier in this chapter.

We're always sure to make a celebration out of answered prayers that we've mentioned as a family. Your children will begin to see and appreciate God's active hand in your family's life as He answers prayers and you rejoice. It's important to teach our children not to take God's blessings for granted but to praise Him in thanksgiving when He touches your life with answered prayer.

How to Teach Your Children to Pray

The number one way you can teach your children to pray is through your example of prayer. They should pray with you and see or hear you pray often. Beyond that, there are a few other things that I believe are helpful. Teach your children the three parts of prayer we talked about earlier in this chapter—praise, petition, and thanksgiving.

When you praise with them, sing some songs that are age-appropriate for them. Younger kids' songs are fun and have catchy tunes. Don't praise and worship with too many songs they are unfamiliar with or to which they don't know the words. And make it fun and enjoyable to them! It might even help to get up and move around, dance, and laugh as you praise God. When you worship, don't let it go beyond their ability to comprehend. As your children grow and mature, they will also mature in their relationship with God, which will also help them grow more intimate with God.

It's important to allow your children to pray from their hearts. Sometimes the way they say something may seem humorous and a little odd to you, but listen to their hearts more than their words.

I fondly remember hearing the story about one of my nephew's prayers when he was around five or six. Each night as he and his brother went to bed, their parents took time to pray with them. One night as he prayed, he began to thank God for protecting them. His prayer went something like this: "God I thank you that you protect us. I thank you that if a big cannonball came flying at me, hit me in the chest, went straight through me, left a big giant hole and hit the wall behind me that you would still be there to protect and heal me." You can imagine the struggle his parents had controlling their laughter. Of course his prayer was humorous and a little odd, but listen to what his heart was saying—he was showing that he believed that God would be there even in extreme circumstances.

Children have a remarkable ability to believe. In fact, we are told to have faith as a little child. Remember our Scripture where Jesus told the disciples not to send the children away? Luke 18:16,17 (NLT) says,

> *Then Jesus called for the children and said to the disciples, 'Let the children come to me. Don't stop them! For the Kingdom of God belongs to such as these. I assure you, anyone who doesn't have their kind of faith will never get into the Kingdom of God.'*

Don't thwart your children's simple faith. Maturity will fix the details. And if something is too far-fetched, gentle correction and seeing their heart will be better than a rebuke.

One mom told me of how her four-year-old son wanted to pray for Superman every night. How cute is that? I told her that at least he was praying for the right side! He could have wanted to pray for one of Superman's arch enemies. I also told her she should gently remind her four-year-old that Superman is pretend and to encourage him to pray for those people who are real too. Listen to his heart, though; he wants the good guy to win, and he wants the bad guys to lose. That sounds pretty good to me. Remember, your children are children; listen to their intentions more than their words as they pray.

> *Your children are children; listen to their intentions more than their words as they pray.*

If you have children who don't know what to say, then give them the words to say at first. When your children were first developing their language skills, you taught them what things were by giving them the words. In the same way, we can teach our children the words they need in order to pray to God. If your example of prayer is not enough, have them repeat after you. Soon they will be ready to try it on their own because you've given them the words.

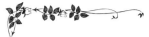 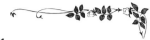

Chapter Six

You Are a Cheerleader!

David and Roxanne Swann say, "You are your child's biggest fan and their loudest cheerleader!" in their book, *Guarantee Your Child's Success*. I love that statement! Nobody should cheer louder for your children than you do.

Your children *want* to please you and have your acceptance, and nothing motivates them toward positive behavior and right choices more than your encouragement. Your encouragement will cause your child to want to continue pleasing you and to actually enjoy being with you. This even works for teenagers!

Let's look at encouragement. Here's my own definition, based on breaking the word down and from its root, *courage*: "To bring into a state of mind whereby one can, with firmness and without fear, stand strong in one's beliefs, even in the face of adversity or challenges." Your encouragement and positive attitude can do all that for your children!

Imagine something as simple as encouragement doing all that for our children. Or is it so simple? To be an encourager, you have to be able to see the positive. You must train yourself to look for the positive in any situation, and unfortunately, most of us have not or do not do this. So that is where we must begin.

We need to change our way of looking at things, to renew our minds and thoughts. Renewing your mind begins with your initial commitment to God through His Son Jesus. Continually allowing the Word of God to change our thought processes is a decision we make every day.

If you are going to encourage your children, you must begin by changing the way you look at things so that you are realistically positive. You must renew your mind. Romans 12:2 says, *"Do not conform any longer to the pattern of this world, but be transformed by the renewing of your mind. Then you will be able to test and approve what God's will is—his good, pleasing and perfect will."*

From that point it is a choice, too. You must continually choose to allow the Word of God to change your thought processes every day. We decide to walk after the leading of the Spirit of God—or not to. If you are sincere in wanting to change your way of thinking from one of complaining, negativism, and defeat to one of overcoming, first make the quality decision to change and then ask the Holy Spirit to help you. Notice how *you* make the decision first. The Holy Spirit cannot work in your life if you do not cooperate.

You can love God because He first loved you, but now the decision is in your hands. You have to *decide* to ask the Holy Spirit to help you, and you have to *decide* to cooperate with Him and change your ways to those of one who overcomes. However, it takes time to change your old ways of thinking. It can sometimes be difficult to begin looking for opportunities to praise your children, but it is worth the effort.

Encouraging your children is similar to preventative maintenance on your car. Most of us start our cars and drive them without giving much thought about how or why they work. But that lasts only as long as the car is running smoothly; when something goes wrong, it gets our attention.

I blew up the engine in the first brand-new car I owned after only one year because I did not take time to change the oil and maintain it properly. It was getting me where I needed to go, and everything seemed to be going along fine—until one day I put the key in the ignition, turned it, and nothing happened. Now the car had my undivided attention, and I, unfortunately, had my husband's attention also. If I had given it a little encouragement to work properly by changing the oil every so often, I wouldn't have had to spend so much time and money fixing it when something went wrong.

A car is an inanimate object. Children are not. They are living, breathing creations of God. Most parents don't recognize good behavior because we are just thankful to have the peace and quiet. But let a storm break out, and they get our attention. However, I believe that if we spend time praising correct behavior and encouraging our children, we will spend less time quelling those sometimes turbulent kid storms.

Every human being loves to be recognized and praised. We respond positively to encouragement and acceptance, and we make a point of going where we receive it. The more we receive, the harder we work to get it. This is not a bad thing. After all, we are made in the likeness of our Father God, and where does He live? In the praises of His people (Psalm 22:2)! The more we praise, the more He dwells with us.

Colossians 3:21 (NKJV) says, "*Fathers, do not provoke your children, lest they become discouraged.*" Ephesians 6:4 (NKJV) echoes this comment: "*And you, fathers, do not provoke your children to wrath, but bring them up in the training and admonition of the Lord.*"

The word *provoke* literally means, "to stir up, arouse, incite, or stimulate," and in both of these Scriptures, it has a negative connotation. The Word of

God specifically tells us to not do things that discourage our children; evidently we should be encouraging them. Hebrews 10:24 in the King James puts a different spin on provoking, however: *"And let us consider one another to provoke unto love and to good works."*

Encouragement adds to your children. When we do things that provoke discouragement in our children, we are subtracting from them and not adding. Encouraging your children has an eternal effect on them! We need to be thinking of ways to encourage them to love and good deeds.

Encouraging your children helps them overcome instead of being defeated. It helps them to defeat the enemy and makes his weapons falter against them so they can lead victorious lives. God encourages (2 Corinthians 7:5), so we, as spiritual representatives of Him through our leadership, need to encourage our children so that when they face adversity and challenges they will have the faith, fortitude, and mental strength to stand and fight.

Some Common Ways We Discourage

◆ **Unrealistic expectations**

We set our children up for failure when we expect something of them they cannot do. Don't purposefully place your children in situations they are not ready or able to handle. Things as simple as asking a preschooler to sit still for long periods of time in church, at a restaurant, or at a social function or expecting your teenager to use the same reason and logic your life experience has given you will discourage them. That isn't to say we shouldn't challenge them to become better and to grow, but you must have correct expectations and handle their failures with grace and care.

◆ **Unclear expectations**

Closely related to unreasonable expectations, not defining the expectations you have for your child's behavior or putting your child in an unfamiliar setting without instruction is an invitation for almost certain failure. Children need to know what you expect of them, and I personally believe in proactive parenting. That means that you need to use your experience, wisdom, and discernment to predict how your child might react in a given situation. And then instead of *re*acting, you instruct them *pro*actively—before the event. You can prepare your children to enter into unfamiliar situations so they don't totally blow it, embarrass you, or worse, embarrass themselves. Children need boundaries, and it is discouraging when they learn that you could have prevented them from messing up but failed to give them the information they needed.

◆ **Nagging**

Nagging accomplishes absolutely nothing! Many people don't understand what real nagging is. Nagging is harping on an issue or when you continuously badger someone past the point where it is beneficial. Nagging comments are often words that we say without purpose and meaning. Your children must really hear your words if you want them to obey you, and human beings have a knack for shutting out nagging. You can't encourage your children if they have stopped listening to you. Do you remember the voices of adults in Charlie Brown cartoons? That is all a person hears who has been nagged too much—nothing but indistinguishable noise in the background.

◆ **Not accepting them for who they are**

God made each one of us unique. Trying to change the core of who God made your children to be discourages them. This is why it is important to pray for guidance as to what path God might have for your child. You must be careful not to try to recreate yourself in your children and to let them be the people God intends for them to be. We need to train and mold our children, but we cannot try to completely change the core of who God created them to be. It's important to learn how to build upon your children's strengths rather than focusing on their weaknesses. If your child has lots of personality and is Mr. or Miss Entertainment, don't try to make them bookworms— mold their natural gifts productively. Learn to celebrate their enthusiasm. If you insist your children be something God did not create them to be, you are training them to be hypocrites and untrue to themselves.

◆ **Not admitting fault**
You are fooling yourself if you think your kids don't know when you've messed up. They usually know it before you do! It's incredibly frustrating when someone wrongs us and then goes on as if nothing happened; don't do that to your children in pursuit of the aura of infallible command. When you do something wrong, admit it and ask for their forgiveness. It will be a tremendous example for them to follow! These can be good opportunities to encourage humility and to model being teachable.

Ways to Encourage—The Importance of Words

The words we speak about and to our children can pierce them like a sword or bring health and healing to them (Proverbs 12:18). It is easy to say things we really do not mean in moments of frustration. Once again, we must change our way of thinking, which in turn will change our actions. The third chapter of the book of James reminds us just how powerful our tongue is. He compares it to the small rudder of a large ship; despite strong winds and the weight of the ship, the small rudder can completely change its course. He says it is also like a small spark that sets a whole forest on fire.

> *Be careful that the words that come out of your mouth bring life to those who hear them—especially your children.*

Our words set the courses of our lives and the lives of those that hear them—especially your children. Proverbs 10:11 says, *"The mouth of the righteous is a fountain of life, but violence overwhelms the mouth of the wicked."* The New Living Translation puts it slightly differently: *"The words of the godly lead to life."* Be careful that the words that come out of your mouth bring life to those who hear them.

One of the ways we can help ourselves to speak only words of life is to look at what Wisdom has to say about her words. Look at Proverbs 8:6-8. This is Wisdom's call to us: *"Listen, for I have worthy things to say; I open my lips to speak what is right. My mouth speaks what is true, for my lips detest wickedness. All the words of my mouth are just; none of them is crooked or perverse."*

Wisdom only says those things that are worthy of saying, and that are right, true, and just. If wisdom is to live in and work through us, we must follow her example. Saying destructive things to our children instead of making constructive statements is not operating in wisdom.

Here are some examples of destructive things I've heard parents say to their children.

- **I am so sick and tired of you!**

  You may be sick and tired of the whole parenting thing at that moment, but are you genuinely sick and tired of your *child*? If you are, please get help. This is not something worthy of saying; it isn't going to change anything to make it better.

- **How stupid can you be?**

  Do you really want the answer to this question? I don't think so; people are capable of nearly boundless stupidity, but there is no value in asking this question because there is no real answer. Asking this is not fair or just either. This type of question only discourages your children because it demeans them and is a negative confession.

- **You're going to be a good-for-nothing all your life.**

  Any statement that is contrary to the Word of God is incorrect and untrue. Wisdom speaks what is right (correct) and true. God has plans to prosper us, give us hope and a future. How *dare* we say anyone is good for nothing when He has such grand plans? People that speak things such as this over their children desperately need to change their thinking; they are going to create that negative reality in their child's life.

- **You can't do anything right; just let me do it!**

  Once again this is an untrue statement. It usually comes from our own frustrations or impatience. Your children can do things correctly, especially when they have been instructed how to do them. If they aren't doing it right, they either aren't ready or haven't been properly instructed—and that's your fault, not theirs. God's Word says we can do all things when we do it with His strength (Philippians 4:13).

*   **Are you going to be a moron your whole life?**

    Well, we certainly hope not, but if this is an example of how you speak to your children maybe they *will* grow up to be morons.

*   **I wish I'd never had you.**

    This is one of the most unfair, unjust statements you can make within the hearing of your children—or beyond it. They didn't ask to be born; again, that's a result of your decision. Your natural actions and God's consequent action of putting the breath of life and purpose in them brought them to earth. Your children's behavior didn't develop in a vacuum, either; they probably learned it from you or you didn't prevent them from picking it up elsewhere with proper discipline.

    I can understand having regrets over the circumstances surrounding the conception of a child or being overwhelmed by the responsibilities of parenting, but please resist the urge to blame the child for those feelings!

    This kind of statement has only one effect—it makes the child feel devalued and crushes their self-esteem and spirit. Proverbs 18:14 says, *"The human spirit can endure a sick body, but who can bear it if the spirit is crushed?"* A child can probably handle physical abuse better than the spiritual wounds statements like these cause. Proverbs 15:13 (NLT) says, *"A glad heart makes a happy face; a broken heart crushes the spirit."*

*   **You are _____**

    Fill in the blank. A liar, a mean child, rebellious, or any number of negative labels we often hear. Be careful not to label your child something they are not. You can speak something over them, causing them to become the very thing you're accusing them of being! Children will exhibit certain behaviors from time to time as they grow through their stages of development. We have to be careful we don't plant them in that stage by the words we speak.

Correct your children's behavior, but do not confess that as being the sum total of their personalities. We correct and discipline for lying, being mean, or being rebellious because we don't want our children to *become* those things. We stop Johnny or Sally from lying so they won't become liars. We stop them from being mean or rebellious so they won't become mean, unkind, or rebellious adults.

It is not true that Junior is a liar just because he told a lie. Have you ever told one? Should we now label you as a liar? Is the word *liar* now part of our description of you? To some, I may be splitting hairs here; and yet we often believe what we hear about ourselves, and a man is what he believes or thinks in his heart (Proverbs 23:6).

The words we say to our children should be positive words and not words that tear them down. Even when we must correct and discipline them, we can use words that motivate them toward right choices and behaviors and not words that belittle them for the wrong they've done. Let me give you an example.

One afternoon, you get a call from your son's school. Johnny has gotten in a fight, and they need you to come to the school right away and take him home. You are really steamed. You wonder how many times are you going to have to talk to him about using self-control. You have a couple of choices here in how you will respond:

Choice #1

You get Johnny in the car and really tear into him. You say everything you feel like saying without regard to the consequences of your words: "I'm so sick and tired of you and your stupidity. You embarrass me on a regular basis! What's wrong with you? I just don't know what to do with you!"

Now, all of this may be true to you at the moment. You very well may be tired of dealing with your son's frequent fights. And obviously if you've had to go to the school and pick him up, you're probably embarrassed. And last, you may not know what else to do at the moment, but throwing all these frustrations into the air within Johnny's hearing may say something to him you don't really mean.

> ಎడ್
>
> *The words we say to our children should be positive.*

Choice #2

What You Said	What He Heard
◆ "I'm so sick and tired of you..."	◆ I don't like you and wish you weren't here anymore.
◆ "...your stupidity."	◆ You are just plain stupid and incapable of intelligent thought.
◆ "You embarrass me..."	◆ I am ashamed you are my son.
◆ "I don't know what else..."	◆ You're a lost cause.

You get Johnny in the car and let him know in no uncertain terms just how displeased you are with his choices and behavior. Remembering you are modeling controlled anger in front of him, you say, "Son, I'm very angry with you right now. You acted very poorly today, and I would be lying if I said I wasn't disappointed by your behavior. There are going to be consequences for what you did today. I'm not sure what yet, but trust me; this kind of behavior will not go unnoticed. Before we get to that, though, let's talk about why you did what you did and how you think you could have and *should have* acted." I hope you can see the differences between the two.

Here is what Johnny is hearing from you in the second example. When you say, "I'm very angry with you right now," Johnny hears that he messed up and you are mad at him for what he did, not for who he is. When you tell him, "You acted poorly," he knows that what he did was wrong. By making sure he knows that you found his *behavior* disappointing, you help him know that you're dissatisfied with what he did rather than who he is. When you inform him there are going to be consequences for his behavior, he will begin to understand that he has to take responsibility for his actions. And last, as you discuss why he did it, you not only help him understand that you care about what he thinks and feels, you can get an impression of the cause of his behavior. This will often help you deal with it more constructively and proactively in the future.

It's important to notice that even when we are angry and frustrated with our children, the words we speak can be gracious and kind—but not wimpy or without conviction. And I'm not saying you should never change the tone of your voice or that everything you say should be soft and flowery.

Proverbs 15:1 says, *"A gentle answer turns away wrath, but a harsh word stirs up anger."* When you respond to your children harshly, they will usually respond in anger. The word *wrath* in this verse originates from a word meaning, "a wall of defense." It's easy to see that your angry response can make your children defensive instead of correcting them, but more importantly, we can often operate out of our own defensiveness and embarrassment. When we're wrathful in our response because we're embarrassed or defensive, we are sowing that into our children. And we reap what we sow.

Instead of making your children defensive by reacting out of your anger, you should encourage them. That doesn't mean you don't correct, but the way you correct is important. Proverbs 16:24 says, *"Pleasant words are a honeycomb, sweet to the soul and healing to the bones."* This Hebrew word for *pleasant* means "agreeable or suitable." In other words, this verse is saying that suitable, appropriate words will bring someone strength or increase—encouragement.

It is important to establish your children's character. Their character is the foundation for their integrity, and it is the key element of successful living. It is important to understand that your children's character and integrity form the underlying structure of their lives. Character is your emotional skeleton—the bones of your life. Your body's bones support and strengthen it, providing attachment points for muscles and tendons as well as protecting your vital organs; character acts in a similar fashion for your life.

When your bones break, you must stop, set them, and take time for them to heal. When your children need aspects of their character fixed, we must stop, pay attention to the problem, and then administer healing. "Pleasant" words will not only taste better going down, they will bring healing, and therefore strengthen the very core or structure of the hearer—in this instance your kids.

When you correct without discouraging your children, it not only goes down better, it will help heal their character breaks. And we have learned that the point where a bone has been broken and mended is actually *stronger* afterward. When you help build and heal your children's character, you are making their lives stronger. In talking about the virtuous wife, Proverbs 31:26 (NLT) says, "*When she speaks, her words are wise, and kindness is the rule when she gives instructions.*" Correct your children and build their character with wisdom and kindness.

Sometimes it doesn't seem "kind" to correct your children at all, but it is far kinder to correct them now, while they are developing, than to leave them alone. Correcting them now prepares them to succeed and not fail in their endeavors. Instruction will encourage your children in the end.

It is important to teach your children the little mannerisms of polite individuals: teach them how to answer the phone and take messages, how to greet someone to whom they are introduced, and how to behave at social events such as weddings, funerals, and dinner at someone else's house. Tell them what is expected of them in these and countless other situations, and give them what I call a "minivision." Set the direction and boundaries for each particular situation. They will form the foundation of their behavior from your instructions, and it will last them their whole lives. Keep their age in mind in your instructions, but it is never wrong to plan for their future. Tell them what you expect in advance: it's very frustrating to learn the rules only after you've begun the "game."

As an example, my children wanted to answer the phone from an early age, so I told them that if they wanted to answer the phone, they first had to learn how. I bought an inexpensive play phone and we practiced. Once they had mastered answering the phone in play, we would let them answer the phone when we gave them permission. They were so polite and gracious that we received many compliments, and it was because they knew what to do and how to do it.

Knowing what is appropriate for their age and personality is also important. We wanted our children to know how to meet new people properly, so we began to teach them how to handle introductions and new people. Dr. Lester Sumrall, a spiritual father to us and a man we considered our pastor, was coming to visit our church, and of course we wanted our children to greet him politely and respectfully when we introduced him to them. I spent the two or three weeks prior to his arrival preparing them for the task.

When the day came and we introduced our children, my husband introduced our gracious and thoughtful daughter, Meredith, first. She very politely walked over to Dr. Sumrall and said, "Good evening. I'm so glad to meet you, Dr. Sumrall." Her father and I beamed at her success. Next came our wonderful, energetic, three-year-old son. My husband said, "Dr. Sumrall I would also like you to meet our son, Stephen Michael." At this, our son broke into a huge smile and a huge *run* all at the same time. He *bolted* across the room, jumped into Dr. Sumrall's lap, and gave him an enormous hug! Dr. Sumrall loved it!

Teach politeness and respect, but remember that three year olds will be three year olds—and Stephen will be Stephen. His greeting of Dr. Sumrall was completely appropriate for a three-year-old and especially for him. That is his personality.

Here is a big one: *always be consistent*. Behavior is conditioned, and you must set consistent standards if you want your children to learn. When you train your children about how they are to act at the store or at Grandma's house, make sure you let them know you *always* expect that type of behavior. Don't be arbitrary in when you instruct them or when you enforce it, and make sure you can and are willing to enforce any behavior that you tell your kids you expect of them.

We have already discussed that your children crave your approval. Your words communicate that you value and approve of them. Approval and validation qualify your children to be the people God created them to be, and when something has been qualified, it has been deemed suitable and proven able. Our words will not only tell our children there is greatness inside of them but also encourage them to live up to that greatness.

⮞∾⮜

Here is a big one: always be consistent.

They will begin to believe they are able to live up to the greatness God has created in them.

It's important to value your children's dreams and the power of their imaginations. If they dream they are someone big—heroic firefighter or famous ice skater—tell them you believe in them and that you can see them doing something as wonderful as being a fireman or an ice skater. Don't be too quick to tell them it's silly or ridiculous!

If your children love to make people laugh, tell them you love their sense of humor and you are proud when they make people happy by being funny. Teach them when it is appropriate, but don't stop them from being free to be who they are. I believe with all my heart that encouraging children this way leads to adults who are not afraid to go after their dreams and will, in turn, accomplish great things with their lives.

In the story of Queen Esther, we read about a young girl who was suddenly taken from an average Hebrew home—a home where she was obviously loved and taken care of by her Uncle Mordecai. Esther finds herself in a foreign environment and faced with the responsibility of saving not just a few people but *her entire nation!* She doesn't believe she is qualified for the task and fears for her own life. Her Uncle Mordecai doesn't become fearful with her; instead he speaks to the greatness in her and reminds her that God has ordained that she be where she is, that she was born for this moment in time. Suddenly she feels qualified and in the end, not only does she save her nation, she and her Uncle Mordecai are given great authority in the king's house.

Paul often spends large portions of his letters encouraging members of the various churches, by reiterating his confidence in their ability to do the right thing or because they have done the right thing.

God has qualified us; now we must agree with His Word over us and repeat what He says to our children. When doubts and fears arise, speak the validating, life-giving Word of God to your children. Read them Psalm 139 and remind them that they were fearfully and wonderfully made.

Remind them that even Paul said he was a competent minister only because God had made him so (2 Corinthians 3:5). It wasn't anything Paul had done; it was the Spirit of God working through him. They are destined for greatness in God's Kingdom not because of what they have done or will do; they have great destinies because of who they are in Christ! Philippians chapter 3 and 4:13, Proverbs 3:26, and Ephesians 3:20 are also great Scriptures for encouraging yourself and your children.

The very thought of my children positively influencing their world excites me beyond words! I hope it does the same for you.

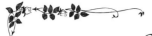 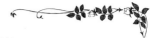

Chapter Seven

Response-Able

Being responsible means that you are trustworthy, in charge, are in authority and are answerable for your actions and/or the actions of others. Wow! That's a lot! Giving your children responsibility is another way to encourage them. It makes them "response-able"—as you give them greater and greater responsibilities and put them in charge of more tasks, they will grow to be more *able* to perform duties. When you train your children to handle responsibility, you're setting them up to be effective leaders in whatever circumstances they find themselves.

Being responsible is not just about learning how to clean a bedroom or take out the trash. It is about teaching kids to think, and it throws off the "I can't" mentality and replaces it with one of confidence and an attitude of diligence. They may not always like this form of encouragement, but it is good for them to learn to set and accomplish goals, to persevere, to be self-disciplined, to feel independent, and to accomplish their ambitions. All of this yields confidence and a healthy self-esteem.

There are many Scriptures in the Bible about being responsible and diligent. Proverbs 12:24 (NKJV) says, *"The hand of the diligent will rule, but the lazy man will be put to forced labor."* Proverbs 21:5 (NKJV) says, *"The plans of the diligent lead surely to plenty, but those of everyone who is hasty, surely to poverty."* 2 Thessalonians 3:10 (NLT) tells us plainly why it's good to teach our children to be diligent when it says, *"Whoever does not work should not eat."* If we never give our children responsibility or something for which they are in charge, they will never experience the satisfaction of a job well done. And they won't understand that success in anything comes from diligence, responsible behavior, and old-fashioned hard work. Without seeing things through responsibly, our children won't understand that success doesn't always come as quickly as we would like it.

Teaching Responsibility

Most successful families function with a teamwork attitude. That means that each member of the family understands that he or she each has a role to play on the team; and when they understand what their position is and play their position well, they contribute and are an integral part of the family's success.

I believe that if we emphasize the importance of teamwork to our children, it will help our homes to run smoothly and more efficiently. Help your children understand that keeping their room clean or taking out the trash is part of their role in helping the family team play the game of life successfully. This has two main benefits: the first is that no one family member needs to be overwhelmed with responsibilities, and the second is that everyone likes to be a part of something successful, and when your children participate, they can share in the benefits of the family's success.

This isn't always easy because, as you may or may not already know, most children seem to think work is a deadly disease. With patience and consistency, teamwork can happen in your home.

Be aware of your children's level of understanding and capabilities before you begin to assign them household responsibilities. If you assign a child a task they are not yet able to accomplish, you will frustrate them, and that will have the opposite effect of what you are working toward.

When our daughter was about four or five years old, I sent her to her room to pick up the toys that were cluttering the entire bedroom floor. I failed to give her proper instruction in how to do this. I assumed she would just go in there and put the toys on the shelf or in the toy box. I also assumed that because she had seen me do it and even helped me do it, she could do it alone.

What I didn't realize was that she was completely overwhelmed by the task I had assigned her. I told her again to put her toys away, but she was getting nowhere. My husband happened to walk by the door and saw her sitting in the middle of the bedroom, moving toys around but not putting them away and looking somewhat forlorn. He asked her what she was doing and why she looked so sad. She told him that I had asked her to put all the toys away, but that she didn't know where to start.

Unlike me, he gave her some help. He explained to her when you have a big job to do, it helps to break it down into little jobs. He asked her where all the stuffed animals went and, of course, she knew. So he told her to put all the stuffed animals away and then come find him and he left the room. A couple of minutes passed and she came running down the hallway asking what she should do next. Step by step, he led her through the process of cleaning up her toys all by herself.

She was so proud of herself when she was done! She made us go in and look at how she had put everything in its special place. A few things she had decided to put somewhere different from where we usually put them and was so anxious to tell us why she thought they fit there better.

It's important to pay attention and not make assumptions about our children's level of understanding and ability. She *was* capable, she just needed some help. We need to stay available to help them when they need more instruction.

If you assign them a job, be sure they understand how to do the job. One of the challenges that you may encounter is "know-it-all" kids. If you begin to give directions and you hear, "I know. I know how to do it," then ask your children to explain to you exactly how they would go about doing the task. You may be surprised to find out they really do know how, or you may find out they don't, despite what they said. If they don't, then tell them there is another way you would like the job done and insist they listen to your directions. Make sure they follow through with your instructions, and don't settle for less than what you have determined they are capable of doing.

Teach them in small steps they can comprehend and take on by themselves. And above all, demonstrate the process and walk them through it a few times before you send them off on their own. In other words, train them for the task. Please also keep in mind that a proper attitude and level of respect should be maintained as well—by both of you! Our goal as parents should always be to set our children up for success and not failure.

If your want your children to begin to make their bed in the morning, don't demand or expect perfection right away. Begin by showing them how to pull the sheet and bedspread up. When they attempt it alone, be satisfied with their effort, even if the bed linens are all wrinkled and crooked. Praise their effort and thank them for helping and being responsible for their own bed.

When you first ask them to help with the dishes, don't start by giving them the dirtiest pots and pans in the house. Give them nonbreakable dishes that are not too dirty so that way they will succeed and not fail. Once again, if the dishes are not as spotless as you could have gotten them, but they are clean, praise the effort. Remember and understand that children—especially young children—don't see things as you do.

They look at the bed they have just made and see perfection—they see accomplishment. You look at it and see a crooked bedspread. As they grow physically, so will their ability to get those linens straight on the bed and those dishes spotless—and so will their desire to get it right. They need to feel pride in their accomplishments.

Demonstrate the task for them and talk them through how to do it, and then let them try. If their attempt is not quite as good as you would like it done, don't redo it in front of them. Let it go. If it bothers you too much, then go back and do it later when they aren't around. They will benefit in the end from believing they did a good job. The sense of

They will benefit in the end from believing they did a good job.

accomplishment they gain builds confidence and a good feeling of worth. As they get older, of course, we must expect more of them and the standard will move up a level.

As children mature in their level of responsibility you should begin to focus on teamwork and leadership. Give them jobs with greater responsibilities and promote leadership in them.

For example, instead of having them *help* with dinner, eventually put them *in charge* of making dinner. Let them decide what to serve and to cook the whole meal.

Have them enlist other family members in the preparations in the same way you would!

The first few attempts may result in interesting meals but in the end, it will be worth it. The benefits outweigh any of the inconveniences. They will be learning to plan and organize, delegate, life skills such as cooking and healthy eating, teamwork, time management, strategizing, and sometimes even problem solving.

Give them the responsibility of managing the yard work, or let them do the grocery shopping one week.

I can imagine the roars of laughter coming from parents as I write this, but I'm serious. I can almost hear you saying, "There is no way on God's green earth I'm letting Junior do the grocery shopping. We'd have nothing but junk food to eat!"

I understand your skepticism; I have two children myself. Please have an open mind and understand that if you prepare your children properly to handle these kinds of responsibilities, they will almost always live up to your expectations. I'm not talking about giving this kind of responsibility to your five-year-old, but if your sixteen-year-old insists he's old enough to drive, then certainly he should be old enough to handle the grocery store or dinner.

Parents set the expectation level, not children. We set it, and we make sure they live up to it. Our training makes them "response-able." The more experience we give our children in being responsible, the more able they will become to handle all kinds of situations!

This produces confident children. This way, even if they are confronted with something they are unfamiliar with, the confidence, self-discipline, perseverance, and diligence you have taught them will carry them through. They will feel and believe they are *able to respond* to whatever task people give them. If you take the time to train your kids to be responsible now for simple things, they will carry the skills, experience, and wisdom gained from that into adulthood and will be an incredible employee, boss, and parent someday.

Let's look at the word *diligence* for a moment. Refer back to the Scriptures in Proverbs earlier in the chapter if you'd like; they're excellent examples.

Diligence is one of the keys to success in any area of life. Diligence places us in leadership positions, makes us rulers—not necessarily over people, although that may happen too, but over life in general. If we are diligent with our finances, we won't find ourselves overdrawn at the bank and charged to the limit on our credit cards. If we are diligent in taking care of our bodies, we won't find ourselves overweight and winded from walking up a flight of stairs. If we are diligent in the training of our children, we will see them grow into powerhouses for the Kingdom of God.

The word *diligence* in Proverbs 10:4; 12:24, 27; and 13:4 is the Hebrew word *charuwts* or *charuts*. Its literal meaning is "incised, incisive, to dig (as in a trench or gold mine) a threshing-sledge (having sharp teeth) and figuratively it connotes determination, eagerness, decision, gold, pointed things, sharp, threshing instrument, wall."

Proverbs 10:4 says, "*Lazy hands make a man poor, but diligent hands bring wealth.*" Proverbs 12:24, 27 (NKJV) says, "*The hand of the diligent will rule, but the lazy man will be put to forced labor.... The lazy man does not roast what he took in hunting, but diligence is man's precious possession.*" Proverbs 13:4 (NKJV) says, "*The soul of a lazy man desires, and has nothing; but the soul of the diligent shall be made rich.*"

Okay, now let's apply this definition to this Scripture and those we read earlier in the chapter. Have you ever used a hoe or other sharp instrument to dig away at something? The more consistently and determinedly you dig the quicker the trench is made. One of the little annoyances of digging a trench is the amount of dirt that falls back into the hole with each strike of the hoe or shovel. The drier and softer the soil, the more of a problem this becomes. It can bring frustration simply because you end up removing some of the same dirt more than once. But diligence, perseverance, and determination will ultimately yield a well-dug trench.

That is why diligent people will find themselves in a position of leadership—because they won't give up and they consistently do what is right. Even when a little dirt falls back into the trench, the diligent person keeps on digging.

As parents, sometimes we will feel as if we are repeating ourselves—digging the same dirt back out of the trench again. Continually repeating the same instructions and administering discipline for the same things over and over again is tiring, but we must continue on diligently doing what we know is right. That doesn't mean you might not try presenting it in different manners, but it means you don't give up. In Galatians 6:9, Paul writes, *"Let us not become weary in doing good, for at the proper time we will reap a harvest if we do not give up."*

We also should teach our children to do the same. By our example, we show them to keep on keeping on despite temporary setbacks—to be diligent. When we allow our children to be responsible for things in their life, they also learn to take responsibility for their own behavior and actions.

Perhaps you tell Johnny to take the trash out, and instead of putting the trash in the container and securing the lid on top as he was instructed, he throws it in the direction of the container and doesn't bother with the lid. When the neighbor's dog gets a hold of the trash and scatters it all over the yard, who will be responsible for the cleanup? Johnny had better be. It was *his* responsibility.

No amount of lecturing or grounding will teach Johnny to take his responsibility seriously more than going out into the yard and picking up all of that nasty garbage. Taking responsibility for his or her own behavior and actions is the beginning of a child's self-discipline.

Let me end this chapter by saying that I know—believe me, I know—how difficult this part of training your children can be, especially if you are having difficulties with being diligent with responsibilities yourself. It takes a lot of work sometimes to organize a family chore list and even more effort to keep it up and running. Continue to emphasize teamwork, and don't let your little munchkins wear you down.

Taking responsibility for his or her own behavior and actions is the beginning of a child's self-discipline.

Keep the benefits your children will be gaining from learning to live life in a responsible manner in mind. Think of the dilemmas you could have avoided if someone had taken time to train you to be responsible. As always, pray! Pray for strength, courage, and wisdom.

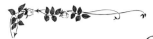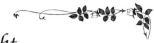

Chapter Eight

Rewards and Bribes

One of the big debates in child-rearing is to pay or not to pay kids for work around the house. I'm not going to resolve this debate here, but I would like to offer a little food for thought in the matter of rewards.

Psychology defines three ways of changing behavior: positive reinforcement, negative reinforcement, and punishment. Positive reinforcement rewards someone for doing a certain action. Negative reinforcement rewards someone for *not* doing a certain action. And punishment takes something away or causes a negative consequence for an action. The first two are encouraging and very valuable for training your child.

Rewards, however, are not bribes, and bribes are nothing like rewards. A reward is something you give after an accomplishment as a way of compensating or celebrating. Bribes are an attempt to influence future behavior and are most often used when dealing with someone who has no moral values. I believe that children should be rewarded for good behavior and for a job well done. I don't believe bribery should be used to motivate them toward good behavior.

Bribes

If you hear yourself saying, "If you will behave yourself in the grocery store, I will buy you a toy on the way home" on a regular basis or if you continually threaten to take away a reward, you have resorted to bribery. You are really saying, "I'm not sure if you are able to behave yourself in an appropriate manner, so I will do *anything* to get you to not embarrass me or make a scene in the grocery store."

Bribes are a temporary means of influencing behavior or attitudes. If you establish this kind of pattern of bribes for proper behavior, you will find that you have to *always* do that each time! Our goal is not to simply control our children *for the moment* but to instill in them proper values and morals. We don't want them to think that each time they do what we want them to do there should be some kind of material reward.

One major problem with this technique for training your children is that bribes start to cost more and more; and even worse than that is the potential for it to turn from bribery to *extortion.* Extortion occurs when someone obtains money or things from someone by threats, oppression, or abuse of authority. If you aren't careful, *your child* will soon have control and will begin to demand things for his or her good behavior. Because you really don't want the little "darling" to embarrass you or make an enormous scene in front of Grandma or your co-worker, you give in to the demand.

I know there is a fine line sometimes between what is a bribe and what is a reward. We need to be aware of what attitude or spirit we are using when we are attempting to motivate our children.

Exodus chapter 23 begins by giving us laws of justice and mercy. One of those laws is, "*Do not accept a bribe, for a bribe blinds those who see and twists the words of the righteous*" (Exodus 23:8). To what does the bribe blind us? It blinds you to the *right reasons* for following the laws or doing the right thing.

The greatest reward we should receive for doing right is knowing that we have honored God with our obedience. The greatest reward our children should receive for doing right is knowing they have honored us with their obedience and thusly honored God. Getting them to this point of understanding is why we use rewards from time to time.

Ecclesiastes 7:7 (NLT) says, *"Extortion turns wise people into fools, and bribes corrupt the heart."* When something is corrupt, it is evil and full of dishonesty. It is also unpredictable. It is unpredictable because it doesn't stem from moral conviction. The highest bidder motivates a corrupt heart, and you won't be able to predict its behavior or know its motivations with certainty.

Children's behavior is unpredictable enough without adding the element of bribery! Proverbs 4:23 says, *"Above all else guard your heart, for it is the wellspring of life."* Jesus says that we will live by what we allow to take root and grow in our hearts, for this is what will come from our mouths (Matthew 12:34, Luke 6:45). Therefore, you must carefully guard your heart—and those of your children.

Remember, a bribe is only a temporary solution to the situation at hand, and in the end it does more to harm the relationship between you and your child than dealing with real behavior issues directly. There may be a few scenes in public or strong battles of the will to begin with, but in the long run, confronting your child's wrong attitudes and behavior directly is a much better way to go.

Rewards

As I stated earlier, rewards are something you give after completing a task or good deed to compensate or celebrate the accomplishment. There are different kinds of rewards and countless ways of dishing out those rewards.

Many adults understand that a job worth doing is a job worth doing well. And most adults understand that not everything we are required to do is pleasant or enjoyable to us. Young children still believe everything in life should be fun and exciting or at the very least something they like. But wonderful tasks such as cleaning a bedroom or doing the dishes are neither fun nor exciting! I'm an adult, and I don't particularly care for doing the dishes and absolutely abhor laundry. My children are learning to do their own laundry early!

Most adults also understand that just because we feel like saying something mean or behaving rudely, it does not mean we can do so. Children are still learning this thing called self-control. So the challenge becomes how to motivate your children to do chores, maintain proper attitudes, and exercise self-control. Before you think, "A good swat on the behind or ground them!" let me offer another suggestion.

We've spent a lot of time talking about encouraging our children. Rewards are another avenue to encourage your kids—reinforcing their good behavior. Rewards are incentives that encourage us to *continue doing* the right thing, not to *get us* to do the right thing. Rewards or incentives should come in both tangible and non-tangible forms.

For example, an allowance based on completed tasks each week is a tangible reward. Allowances are something that should happen weekly, biweekly, or monthly and work similarly to the way your salary works. You get paid based on whether or not you perform the job for which you were hired. When you don't do the job for which you were hired, you aren't paid—at least not for long.

Am I saying children should get paid for everything they do around the house? No! Am I saying you have to use an allowance as a means of reward? No. It is an option and an example for you only, but it will help your kids learn self-control in their finances as well.

Another example might be allowing a friend to sleep over and making it a fun night; that could be a good tangible reward for keeping a room tidy for a whole week or for some other goal. Rent a favorite movie or video game, order pizza, or take them out bowling—let them stay up late having fun being kids! Let it be kid fun night! You know the kind where we don't *have* to do anything or be too scheduled or too quiet.

Here's an idea how to make this work. Put a chart up somewhere visible to both you and your child. At night as you put your children to bed, check the room to determine if they have kept it clean in the manner in which you asked them. If they did, put a check mark on the chart for that day. Let them see you do it and congratulate them for a job well done. Make a big deal out of it. Make it a game to see how many check marks in a row they can get if they want to. Determine ahead of time how many days out of the week your goal is for them.

And don't nag them. Just keep reminding them (in a lighthearted manner) that hard work and clean rooms make dads and moms happy and that happy dads and moms become generous dads and moms.

If they meet the goal you set, then reward them. As your children get older, allow them to set their own goals and work toward accomplishing them.

One idea we used around our house was the Treat Jar. The Treat Jar was a cleaned out mayonnaise jar with a decorated lid. Inside it written on little pieces of paper were fun things like five dollars and a trip to the toy store to pick out anything they wanted. Oh, the ridiculous things they bought with that five dollars! There were also sleepovers (our daughter's favorite), pizza and a movie with a friend, a trip to our local video game store to buy a used video game (our son's favorite), and other fun things for them. When one of our kids would do something we thought deserved celebrating or rewarding, we would get the Treat Jar down and let them pick out a treat. The treats changed from time to time, and we didn't use the Treat Jar for everything. We used this mostly when our kids were very young and for things like showing kindness, sharing, or going the whole day without fighting (a major accomplishment back then).

Don't hesitate to pour sincere praise into your children.

One of the best ways to reward your children is praising them. Praise is non-tangible because it can't be held in your hand at that particular moment, but its effects will follow you throughout your life. Don't hesitate to pour sincere praise into your children. When they obey speedily and cheerfully, tell them loudly and clearly how much you appreciate it! Make a big deal about it every time.

Don't offer your children insincere flattery. We aren't trying to butter them up to get obedience or kindness out of them. Genuine praise encourages them to continue with the hard work or proper behavior they have shown. It also lets them know when they've done something correctly. Be sure to notice even the smallest of improvements, and don't wait for perfection every time.

If Johnny lost his temper but stopped himself from biting Sally, correct him for losing his temper but please praise him for not biting or hitting—especially if aggressive behavior is an issue for him. We had a biter in our house, and it wasn't until I changed my perspective and began to acknowledge the times my child did use self-control that I saw improvements. My anger, frustrations, and embarrassment didn't help, but consistent praise and correction did.

In learning to reward our children, we gain something invaluable as well. We learn to be more optimistic and to look for and see the positive rather than the negative. When I began to look for ways to reward my children, I honestly began to expect them to behave rather than to misbehave. Will it alleviate your need to correct and discipline? No, but amazingly it will change your perspective. Trust me! Try it! It works!

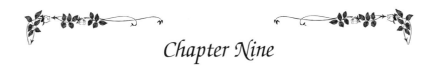

Chapter Nine

The Dynamic Duo:
Honor and Obedience

When parents fall asleep, we don't see sugarplums dancing in our heads; we see well-mannered, obedient children. Children who say, "Yes ma'am," and, "Yes sir," and gleefully skip off to do what we have asked of them. Then, of course, we wake up.

I want you to know that it doesn't have to be a dream. Well-mannered, obedient children are well within the realms of reality—if you are willing to take the time to teach, train and nurture them in that direction. I've titled this chapter *The Dynamic Duo: Honor and Obedience*, because the two must work together. They walk hand in hand.

If I have obedient children but no honor, I have nothing more than slaves. Slaves are not willing servants but people being made to stay somewhere and do work against their own will. Before I go any further, let me say that I believe children should and must learn to obey their parents! In the famous words of Susannah Wesley, mother to John and Charles Wesley and their fifteen siblings, you must "subdue self-will in a child, and thus work together with God to save the child's soul."

Self-will in both children and adults must be taught and trained in order to submit to authority. The first step in subduing self-will is to teach the principle of honoring authority. Let's look at a few Scriptures that will build a foundation for honor.

Exodus 20:12 (NKJV) says, *"Honor your father and your mother, that your days may be long upon the land which the* LORD *your God is giving you."*

> *Children, obey your parents because you belong to the Lord, for this is the right thing to do. 'Honor your father and mother.' This is the first of the Ten Commandments that ends with a promise. And this is the promise: If you honor your father and mother, 'you will live a long life, full of blessing.'*
>
> Ephesians 6:1-3 (NLT)

The first four of the Ten Commandments have to do with our relationship with God. The next six deal with how we relate to each other. Interestingly, the first of these six—the fifth commandment—addresses the parent/child relationship. It is also interesting to note that the commandment does not deal with the action of obedience but the attitude of honor. That is because true obedience comes from an attitude of honor. Obedience naturally follows honor.

In two of the most well-known Scriptures dealing with obedience to parents, found in Ephesians and Colossians, Paul says that obedience is the right thing to do and that it pleases God, but he says *honoring* your parents brings the blessings of God. Many times throughout Scripture, we read references to people honoring God with their lips but not their hearts. That kind of honor is not genuine. It is blatant hypocrisy and nothing but flattery.

True honor is an attitude that flows from the heart and that our actions of cooperation and obedience demonstrate. Attitudes are the way we think and believe about something, and they determine how our life will go. Attitudes are also choices, and we face choices to continue in right attitudes or not every day. It is imperative that we begin to teach and train our children early how to honor us as the direct authority in their lives.

Hebrews 13:17 says, "*Obey your leaders and submit to their authority. They keep watch over your souls as men who must give an account. Obey them so that their work will be a joy, not a burden, for that would be of most advantage to you.*" It's important to teach your children the advantages of choosing to honor and obey those in authority. Don't be afraid to tell your children that they are accountable to God—and often other people—for their actions while they are young.

In teaching your children the principle of honor there are five things of which you must be aware:

1. **You must honor God first.** You honor God by following and delighting in His commandments and Word. You demonstrate this by doing things such as reading your Bible, faithful attendance at church, tithing and giving offerings, exhibiting the fruit of the Spirit in your life, living a life of obedience, and respecting authority God has placed in your life. Children are perceptive. It will be evident to your children whether or not you truly honor God. There is a spiritual aspect to this also; if a true spirit of honor resides in your home, it will begin to transfer into the lives of your children. Unfortunately, the opposite is also true. (See Romans 13:1-5)

2. **Be an honorable person.** Be a person of integrity, a person worthy of honor. You can show this to your children by keeping your word to the best of your ability—especially around your children. Don't be dishonest with them or other people. Pay your bills on time. Don't gossip. If it is necessary to

discuss something negative concerning someone you know, don't do it in front of the children. Don't look for ways to beat the system or new ways to cut corners. Your children will see this and gain a good work ethic.

3. **Teach your children what the Bible says about authority.** Take time to give them examples of people who submitted to authority and the benefits of their honor and submission. People such as David, Abraham, Jesus, his mother Mary, the Roman centurion with the sick servant Jesus healed, and the Apostle Paul are just a few of the many examples you can give them. Give them examples from your own life where you honored authority and were blessed— or instances where you dishonored authority and suffered the consequences of that choice.

> *Give them examples from your own life where you honored authority and were blessed.*

4. **Do not allow your children to speak or act disrespectfully to you or other authority figures.** Remember, people demonstrate true honor through their actions. We have always made it clear to our children they are free to say just about whatever they need to say to us if they can say it with honor and respect. If it can't be said with honor and respect, it doesn't need to be said. If they willfully say something or act without honor or respect, we always discipline them quickly so they understand the relationship. Don't tolerate dishonor in your home at any level, even between you and your spouse.

5. **Do not treat your children disrespectfully.** It is sometimes easy to abuse our authority and use it as an excuse to treat our children without respect. Examples would be when an adult totally disregards their children's feelings, continually gives no thought to their wishes or thoughts, neglects their spiritual, emotional, or physical needs, or speaks to them in a manner that degrades them. It is unacceptable for an adult to get in a child's face and scream at the top of his lungs, especially if that screaming includes foul language and/or sarcasm. It is not a fair fight, so to speak, especially if you then expect *them* to honor *you* after you've just disrespected them. This is a sure way to provoke resentment in your kids. Verbal and physical abuse scar children emotionally in ways that take considerably more effort to repair than it took to create the damage.

Always remember, your example is the strongest teaching and training tool you have. Let a spirit and attitude of honor prevail in you first.

Obedience

It is imperative to teach your children the principle of honoring their parents. It is equally important that they learn to obey you.

I was reading through Deuteronomy one day and came across a few verses that shocked me. Deuteronomy is Moses' farewell address to the children of Israel. In it, he restates the law that God gave him for the Israelites. In Deuteronomy 21:18-21, he tells them what to do with a child who will not obey his parents or respond to their voice.

He tells them they are to take the child to the elders of the city, and to tell them that he is rebellious, reckless, and disobedient. The elders and men of the city were to then stone him to death! Moses considered this kind of behavior evil and not to be tolerated! If the parents had to do this, all Israel was to hear about it and be afraid.

I bet if this was the standard today, we wouldn't have a whole lot of problems with rebellious teenagers. Yikes! Every once in a while when our kids get a little too full of themselves, we remind them how blessed they are to be living under grace and not the Law!

What we should learn from this passage is not that we should resort to stoning our rebellious children but instead to see how important it is for children to listen to us for correction and discipline. Obviously, God takes this pretty seriously. This also lets us know that a rebellious child is not one who just gets into trouble or mischief a lot but one who *makes a willful decision* not to acknowledge, obey, or respond to his parents' voice.

For your children to obey, they must not only hear your words; they must *value* them. The words I say to my children must mean something to them! They should carry a much greater weight than the words their friends or even their teachers speak to them. In other words, children should honor and obey their parents' words.

To accomplish this, here are a few guidelines:

+ Teach your children to obey you the *first time* you say something to them. By doing this, you are beginning to subdue self-will and teaching them that your words have value and must be obeyed promptly. Correct and discipline them for anything less.
+ Teach your children to respond to you before you resort to yelling. Use a conversational tone. Your

tone or intensity may change, but do not get in the habit of having to yell to get their attention.

- Don't allow them to debate their obedience. For those of you who have children that are gifted communicators or early analytical thinkers, this one's for you. Your children will sweep you into a debate faster than you can blink. Sometimes we should take time to explain why we have asked them to do something, if it is relevant to the task and their ability to complete it. Other times, they need to just *obey*. We don't need to discuss terms of obedience or the timeliness of it. Often we understand as we walk out our obedience.

- Don't threaten, bribe, or try to manipulate obedience out of your children. Saying something like, "If you don't come with me right now, I'm going to leave you here at the store," is nothing more than an idle threat and a feeble attempt to manipulate obedience. We've already talked about the consequences of bribery. State your desire clearly and *insist* they follow through.

The objective is to get your children to obey without hesitation, complaints, bad attitudes, or disrespect. My grandmother used to say, "I don't need any back talk; I need some action. Now get to it young lady," and if I didn't get to it fast enough, Grandma's yardstick had a way of speeding things up a bit.

Are there ever any instances when we should make an exception to

⊙∽⬦

The objective is to get your children to obey without hesitation, complaints, bad attitudes, or disrespect.

speedy obedience? Yes. Remember patience and understanding are also working here, too. Take time to make sure that your children understand clearly what it is you have asked of them and how to accomplish it. Remember the story about our daughter cleaning her room? She understood what I had asked her to do but not *how*, and this hindered her ability to obey.

There are a few times when your children honestly might not hear you speak to them. "I didn't hear you," I know, is a classic kid line, and it's sometimes amazing how those kid ears work. Such miraculous selective hearing! To fix this, whenever possible make sure your children are looking you in the face, making eye-to-eye contact, when you are talking to them. Go a step farther if you need to and make them repeat what you have just said to them to *guarantee* they understood. You have just taken away their excuse. I have even occasionally seen a preschooler figure out how this works and attempt to avoid the eye contact thing so as to not be held responsible for his or her behavior! Children never cease to amaze me in their ability to figure things out. But obviously, they can't be allowed to get away with it.

When our son was about six years old, we started to have him take the trash from the kitchen to the garage by himself. One of the first times I asked him to do this, I gave him the bag of garbage and told him to take it to the big trash can in the garage, put it in there, and be sure to replace the lid. He repeated my instructions, picked up the bag and off he went. A little while later I walked by the door leading into the garage and lo and behold the bag of garbage was sitting there by the door, still inside the house. I called him, had him repeat the directions to me, and then asked why the garbage was sitting there if the instructions were to put it in the garage.

I reminded him that it wasn't obedience if he didn't follow the instructions completely. He started to look a little nervous and shuffled his feet. So I asked what the problem was. He said he was scared to go into the garage because he heard a funny noise and when he opened the door he was sure he saw a big dragon.

I know my son—I know when he is trying to fool me and when he is not. He honestly thought there was some creature in the garage making a kind of ticking, buzzing noise! I reassured him that big dragons were only pretend, took him by the hand, and led him into the garage (without the bag of garbage). Together we walked around the garage until we found the source of the noise, which turned out to be the water softener recycling. He had never heard the water softener before and didn't even know what it was. Once I had alleviated his fear, I sent him to get the bag of garbage and complete his chore while I stood in the doorway.

If your child is afraid to do what you have asked him, take a minute and evaluate the situation. Have you asked them to do something that is too hard, or, as in this story, causes them fear? You can usually alleviate their fear by a simple explanation. Follow-up is very important! Don't become so legalistic in your efforts to teach honor and obedience that you don't leave room for children to be children.

Strong-Willed Children

I used to think of a strong-willed child only in terms of being stubborn or belligerent—a child who would argue with you just *because* and who was cantankerous and generally disagreeable. While all of the above may be true to some degree, it all sounds so negative! This kind of child would seem to be a parent's worst nightmare! Call me the starry-eyed optimist if you want to, but let's take a minute and look at it from another angle.

Someone who is strong rather than weak is able to withstand a lot of pressure. Your will is your ability to make decisions; it's your rationale, your reasoning, and your logic.

Wouldn't it be a parent's greatest dream to have a child who has it within him or her to use reason, rationale, and logic to make a decision and then stand by that decision despite great amounts of pressure? I know that the battle with that will can be exhausting to a parent's spirit, soul, and body, but you must keep your eye on the prize—not the fight. Strong-willed children must know that your will is stronger and therefore will prevail when needed. And that's the key—you must prevail when you need to.

The point is not to destroy the child's will but to bring it under your authority. We want to teach all children to willingly submit themselves first to God and then to us. Before children learn to submit to God's will, they must first learn to submit to ours.

Many people have written entire books about strong-willed children, and I am not going to attempt to duplicate their work, but I would like to give you a few highlights and pointers that might be helpful in learning to deal with your children.

Not all strong-willed children are vocal and aggressive in exercising their will. Some are very quietly determined. A quiet, strong-willed child will smile and agree with you at the moment and then go do what they wanted to anyway. This type will catch you off guard because you'll think everything is good and then be surprised to discover they've done the exact opposite.

Then there's the loud aggressive type who will attempt to debate, argue, and negotiate everything to the point where you want to scream at the top of your lungs. In either case, here are four things to keep in mind:

1. **Consistency is key!** This is a tough one, but it is imperative that the *rules stay the same each and every time*. Most strong-willed children I've met are quick thinkers and will discover a loophole immediately. Once they find the loophole, they will not hesitate to start jumping through it. Set the standards; write them down and post them somewhere in your house if you need to; but whatever you do, stick to them no matter what!

2. **Be firm but kind.** When enforcing the rules, be rock solid but tempered with love. Say what you mean, and mean what you say. Don't scream at the top of your lungs. Talk to them with such resolve in your voice that there is no doubt that you will stick to your decision, and then do not argue the point any further. Only allow for discussion of any matter *before* you make a decision—and only if you really think you need or want to allow the child to voice his or her view to help you in making the decision.

3. **Do not lose control** or become overly frustrated with them. When we lose control of a situation, we lose our ability to deal with it effectively. Our minds begin to race, and often we say or do things that do more harm than good. If you are that angry or frustrated, send the child to his or her room—and you go to yours for a few minutes to calm yourself and regain your rationale!

4. **Enlist help** for yourself and for your child if you need it. You are not alone! Many parents and children have gone through what you are going through. Ask someone who is trustworthy, such as your pastor or a reliable friend or relative, or enlist professional help. Don't ask someone whose kids are disrespectful and disobedient! Look for parents whose children are under control. You will be surprised to find out how

many of them will say their children are strong-willed. Most will be more than happy to talk with you. Make sure all those who are dealing with your child on a regular basis know what your standards of behavior are. Let those people know how they can help you and that you are there to help them. I call it an ambush. Just when your strong-willed child thinks he or she is out of sight and can do as they please, surprise attack them with other helpers that can help you uphold your standards of behavior, even when you're not there! My kids really think that somehow we have eyes everywhere. And we do.

Do not give up! I know this may seem obvious, but it goes back to the consistency key. Dealing with a truly strong-willed child will be exhausting in *every* way. Strong-willed children are not that way one day and not the next; they are that way day in and day out. It is their nature, and when it comes for standing for the Kingdom, it will be an invaluable resource to them.

Hang in there. Read everything you can get your hands on about training strong-willed children. And remember; keep your eye on the *prize*—a child whose strong will is set toward Christ—not the fight. In the end, you are going to have a dynamic adult son or daughter who will stand for righteousness and the Kingdom of God with such resolve and determination it will amaze you!

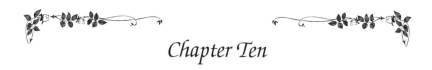

Chapter Ten

Correction and Discipline

You must start with a proper foundation. Before discipline can be effective in your child, you must establish a proper foundation of love. Understanding you have a covenant relationship with your children is a vital key to your foundation for discipline. Your children must believe that you love and accept them unconditionally; then when you must exert your authority over them, it will be effective. If I believe that someone has my best interest at heart and is truly motivated by their love and concern for me, my response to their rebuke or discipline will be different than if I thought they didn't care at all.

God likes proper balance, and Proverbs talks about how God abhors dishonest scales (Proverbs 11:1). The weights and balances of a scale must be set correctly for the scale to give an accurate result. Allow the Word of God to adjust your weights and balances so that you are able to give accurate amounts of both love and discipline.

You'll be out of balance if you give your children unconditional love and encouragement but withhold proper discipline and correction from them. The results of this permissive style of parenting will produce self-centered, arrogant, and/or insecure children.

The same is true for the opposite. If all your children receive from you is discipline and correction but don't understand your unconditional love, the results could be aggressive children or broken children. Generally, those who parent their children in this way are extremely controlling and critical and don't understand what they are taking away from their children.

Your Motivation

Love must be the only motive for correction and discipline. First Corinthians 13:5 reminds us that true love is not self-seeking. Disciplining your child solely because you are angry or embarrassed is not acceptable and will *not* accomplish your intention. As parents, of course, we will from time to time be angry with or embarrassed by something our children do but we cannot allow these things alone to push us into discipline. If we sow anger into our children we will reap anger. What is the bottom-line reason we discipline our children?

The desired goal of correcting and disciplining our children is to teach them to correct and discipline themselves. Teaching them to motivate and control themselves should be foremost in our hearts and minds. We want them to learn to be personally responsible for their actions, aware of how their actions affect others, and to stand on their own merits without needing to compare or contrast with others. Henry Cloud and John Townsend in their book, *Boundaries,* say it this way:

> Discipline is an external boundary, designed to develop internal boundaries in our children. It provides a structure of safety until the child has enough structure in his character to not need it. Good discipline always moves the child toward more internal structure and more responsibility.

Good discipline is not just punishments and penalties for wrongdoing; it also gives correction. It builds something internally in your children. It gives them something to stand on so they have the ability to not make the same mistake again.

When we correct something, we fix it or make it right. Usually we are attempting to correct a way of thinking or lack of understanding. We bring change so something moves from wrong to right or from abnormal to normal. Correcting your child is often verbal and instructive in its nature. Remember, it is not enough for parents to point out the wrong a child has done and punish them for it. We must show our children how to *fix* their mistakes. This is the structure to which Henry Cloud and John Townsend are referring.

Proverbs 22:15 (NLT) says, *"A youngster's heart is filled with foolishness, but discipline will drive it away."* Often the word *foolishness* is interpreted as rebellion, but the word actually means just what is says—foolishness or lack of understanding. Children often do not realize they have done anything wrong until we point it out to them.

I'm reminded of a true story of some children—and one child in particular—who, because of foolishness and poor judgment, managed to empty the entire contents of a *fire extinguisher* in a classroom of a newly completed educational wing at their church! I won't give the name of anyone in the guilty party, mostly so one particular parent doesn't have to hide her head in shame, partly because some people might say that his parents should have been paying more attention. I will say that the culprits were all very nearly taken to the city gates to be stoned—by their own parents! Fortunately for them, we live under grace, but rest assured that at least one certain child learned the error of his ways!

Sometimes our children know exactly what they've done, and other times they simply don't understand that their actions were foolish. When you bring the error of their ways to their attention, you must explain what it was, and why—if you can—it was not appropriate behavior. It's also good to give your children the opportunity to tell how they would fix it or do differently the next time. Many children, when given instruction and a little bit of understanding, will know exactly how to fix it. If they don't, you must help them by telling or showing them how to fix it and by creating an environment that directs them in the correct path.

❧

Sometimes our children know exactly what they've done, and other times they simply don't understand that their actions were foolish.

This environment is an atmosphere of responsibility for their actions and discipline. Sometimes you'll have to make this environment a fairly tight squeeze on them in order to get them heading in the direction they should go.

There are three aspects of discipline I would like to address: training, control, and acceptance.

Training

Proverbs 22:6 says, *"Train a child in the way he should go, and when he is old he will not turn from it."* This is one of the Scriptures parents quote most! To me, it is one of the anchor Scriptures to which parents can cling. When the kids are acting crazy, and we feel as though *we* are going crazy, it is one of the Scriptures parents hold on to for dear life. I would like to take a closer look at this anchor.

The Hebrew word for *train* is *hanak* or *chanak*, and is usually translated as "dedicate, inaugurate, or initiate." Proverbs 22:6 is the only place where this word is translated *train* in the NIV. The intended meaning then is that we begin or set a child on the right course from the beginning and he won't depart from that course as he matures and becomes responsible for his actions.

Webster might say that when we train our children, we are instructing them to make them skillful or capable of doing something, aiming them, or directing them. The training I give my children should cause them to realize they have been set apart for the Kingdom of God and awaken in them the desire to commit themselves to the ways of God. When you dedicate your children to God's ways, you're setting them apart and committing them—and yourself—to a certain cause, course of action, or way of thinking. Further, our instructions and actions should direct and aim them toward the purposes of God for their individual lives as well as make them *feel* skilled and capable.

This sense of godly purpose is very important, because I promise you will be disciplining children more when they don't have a sense of destiny. Children who wander aimlessly because they have no vision or purpose have a tendency to get into trouble.

Proverbs 28:19 says without a vision (a dream, revelation) people perish (are undisciplined, get out of hand). Children and adults alike without vision will, in search of meaning and purpose, often look to things or people rather than the God who created them. Train your children in such a way that you give them a sense of purpose and direction. Speak the Word of God over them, and when correcting or punishing them, keep in mind you are aiming them toward their purpose and not just stopping unwanted behavior.

I've included some Scripture references that you might find helpful. They have many connections between discipline and creating a level, well-lit path for your children to follow.

- Hebrews 12:5-13
- Proverbs 3:11,12
- Proverbs 4:10-27
- Proverbs 5:7-14
- Proverbs 3:18
- Proverbs 23:22-26

- Proverbs 29:1; 17,19
- Proverbs 15:5,10b
- Proverbs 10:17
- Proverbs 12:1
- Proverbs 19:18

Control/Authority

As parents, we have authority over our children. That means we are to keep them under our authority and take responsibility for them and their actions. It is our responsibility to regulate and direct their behavior. We must be the dominating force exerted upon them.

I know this may sound harsh and extremely direct, but, as the cliché goes, sometimes the truth hurts. Parents cannot alleviate themselves of the responsibility of controlling their children. It is not the job of schools, churches, or the local police department to ensure your children are not wreaking havoc on society. If your four-year-old is running through the local discount store tearing clothes off the racks, it is not the responsibility of the store management or security to control him; it is yours.

Gaining control over your children starts early in their lives. It starts by not allowing them to manipulate you or the rest of the family by their tantrums or strong wills. Self-will is at the root of our carnal nature. It is and will always be at odds with our spirit. We must first choose to not allow self-will to rule but bring our flesh under subjection to the Spirit of God, replacing our own spirit as the ruling force in our life. Subduing self-will and bringing it under submission to authority is the only way of ensuring growth, favor, and success in our lives.

Teaching our children to operate in this principle begins by teaching them that their will must be subject to ours. Notice I did not say their will must be destroyed; we are not controlling them in an unhealthy way. Discipline has the ability to create a straight, level, well-lit path that will help your children submit to authority. It creates an environment that causes children to choose to submit because they eventually see the benefits of it.

Acceptance

Children must learn to receive and accept all forms of discipline. Of course they won't like it—who does?— and neither will they thank you for punishing them. No child or adult likes to be rebuked or chastised. But what they like isn't the important thing. It's important that they learn to receive discipline.

Remember, discipline is supposed to teach our children to be *self*-disciplined. We are not looking to simply manage behavior; we are building a foundation within them on which they can build in turn. Our goal is not just for them to go through the appropriate discipline but to benefit from it.

Children must be taught to accept discipline willingly early in their lives. Allowing them to fight against it, verbally or physically, is not acceptable. You must begin to teach your children to accept discipline before they reach adolescence. Begin when they're toddlers; it's not too early. You should never ignore temper tantrums, though these are normal for a toddler or preschooler. It's also important that you don't give the impression to your children that resisting discipline in any way is humorous or acceptable. For instance, it might be funny to watch your toddler try to escape you, but don't communicate it to them—they'll only take that and *run* with it!

Let me relate a story from my own childhood that my parents and I laugh at now and they did then. My parents believed in the rod of correction—otherwise known as spanking. I, of course, did not and would come up with various means of trying to avoid receiving the spanking each time they were about to spank me. I would begin to lavish love on my father or mother, declare my great love for them, suddenly have to go to the bathroom, cry, or declare my innocence and the unfairness being imposed on me.

I also would move as the swats were inflicted, sometimes running in circles causing my father to also run in circles. One day I was in the running mode and while my father ran in circles with me he realized he was getting dizzy. Although the circles I made were large, his were more like spinning around in one spot. Immediately, he realized that a change was needed. From that time on, both my brother and I were made to lie across the bed and be still to receive our discipline. There was to be no more begging, pleading, or running. My father established this policy at the time for practical reasons—his own sanity and safety—but in reality, it was also teaching us to, in a physical sense, be still and receive punishment willingly.

The heart has to be receptive as well. It doesn't mean your children have to enjoy it, but they must learn to receive it. Have you ever had to take horrible tasting cough medicine? Did you enjoy it? Of course not, but you endured it because you knew it would benefit you if you did. Receiving discipline works in much the same way.

Solomon coined thousands of wise sayings, many of which are quoted in the book of Proverbs. He admonished his son to listen to and heed both God's discipline and that of his parents. Many passages convey a real sense of urgency. In Proverbs 23:26, he says, *"My son, give me your heart."* The heart is the seat of our desires; when we give our heart to something, it proves our true intentions, motivations, and desires.

Go after your kids' hearts! Win their hearts and they will know despite all of the unpleasantness they might be experiencing, their parents love them and have their best interest at heart.

Practicalities of Discipline

How do we practically go about disciplining our children? They must learn there are rewards for obedience and good choices and consequences for disobedience and poor choices early. Rewards can be praise, privileges, and greater opportunities; consequences can take the form of confrontation and discipline. They must learn that *they* are accountable and responsible for the rewards and consequences they receive. If your children obey or make good decisions, they should get the full

> *They must learn that they are accountable and responsible for the rewards and consequences they receive.*

credit for their actions. The same applies for the opposite. They need to learn that no one else is accountable for their disobedience or poor decisions. Galatians 6:4,5 says, *"Each one should test his own actions. Then he can take pride in himself, without comparing himself to somebody else."*

Forms of Discipline

Reality Discipline

The easiest form of discipline is what I call "reality discipline." It is simply letting children deal with whatever the natural consequences of their actions require. It is easy if we resist the urge to step in and deflect the consequences or soften the blow. It is in our nature—especially moms—to protect our children from all harm. It is not real life to shelter them from *everything* that could bring them discomfort, though. They must learn there are consequences for their actions.

Let's say that the policy in your home is that your children must do their chores before playtime begins. Your little darling procrastinates and does not pick up her room. The phone rings, and it is one of her friends asking if she can go to a movie and sleep over with some of their other friends. You have a decision to make—stick with the policy or let it slide and have her clean it tomorrow when she gets home. Ask yourself a couple of questions. Is procrastination and ignoring policy a habit with your sweet pea? If not, ask yourself if you are willing to allow it to become a habit. As a general rule, sticking with the guidelines you have established builds more self-discipline than overlooking them.

If Junior lies and is caught in his lie, should he only be disciplined privately or should you make him go to the person to whom he lied, tell the truth, and apologize? Ask yourself which route would build the most self-discipline in Junior. Having to tell the truth and apologize makes him deal *directly* with his wrong action.

One more scenario to consider: Let's say you have told your Pumpkin Pie that she is expected to put her bike away each time she is finished riding it, rather than jumping off it and letting it lay wherever. If she leaves it lying in the driveway and someone backs over it with the car, the natural consequence would be the loss of her bike, correct? Softening the blow of this consequence would be dad and mom running out that weekend and replacing the bike. Fully dealing with the consequences would be Pumpkin Pie having to, through some reasonable means, earn the bike back.

Imposed Discipline

Imposed discipline is discipline that is affected on your child by an outside force—namely you, the parent. Examples would be lost privileges, extra chores, time-outs, repeating an action, physical punishment, or loss of a previously earned reward. Whatever the imposed discipline is, remember, it should be directing your child down the path of building self-discipline in him.

Be creative. Don't always fall back on the old standards of grounding or spanking. For instance, if Johnny has not followed through with your instructions for taking care of the family pets (such as not putting the dog food away properly or not cleaning out the dishes regularly), instead of always grounding him, why not sit down, have an easy discussion on the importance of following directions and then have him write a short essay on the benefits of it? Or take a minute and write out specific instructions for the chore and have your child write a copy or copies of it? If your children are like ours, they feel like they get enough writing assignments through schoolwork and the last thing they want is to write another essay! It can make for effective punishment.

Because we want our children to realize the significance of the Word of God in our lives, we have from time to time also had them copy Scriptures having to do with their offense. We don't present this to them in condemnation but as a reminder of what God has to say about the subject and the importance of following His commands. If used properly, the Word will bring enlightenment and conviction.

Another creative idea to use for bad attitudes would be to make your children repeat their response to an instruction. If I ask one of my children to turn the television or computer off and get busy cleaning their room, I expect them to respond by turning the television off and going to clean their room, all with a proper attitude. Griping and complaining, huffing and puffing, and slamming doors is *not* a proper response. My response to this would be a quick reminder that it is not acceptable for them to behave like that and they can come back and try it repeatedly until we get not only the actions correct but also the attitude.

No discipline is pleasant at the time. Effective discipline *should be* uncomfortable. It should create pressure or stress. It must bring them to attention, strengthen them, and create a level path for them. If it does these things, it will result in a good harvest of righteousness in them. Hebrews 12:11 says, *"No discipline seems pleasant at the time, but painful. Later on, however, it produces a harvest of righteousness and peace for those who have been trained by it."*

Consider the following personal story: By the time our son was preschool age, we were well aware that we were dealing with a wonderfully strong-willed little boy. I, in particular, found myself becoming increasingly frustrated and completely exhausted by his continual stubbornness and uncooperative nature. To put it bluntly, although I loved him dearly, I found myself *not liking him.* I hope you understand the difference.

It was difficult to get up day after day and know the day would be mostly a battle. It seemed as if every discipline imposed was ineffective. He continued to do as *he willed.* One day as I prayed, I asked the Holy Spirit to show me what to do to begin to bring his will under subjection to mine.

Even as I spoke this aloud, I realized my focus had been all wrong. Even though I prayed for the correct thing, I had been focusing on controlling or stopping his undesirable behavior instead of teaching *him* to control or stop *his own* undesirable behavior.

The next time we had a battle of the wills, instead of quickly swatting him on the behind and fussing at him for his behavior, I simply picked him up, sat him on a chair facing the corner, and told him he had to sit there for two minutes. I also told him he would not be allowed to complain or ask me how much longer he had to sit there and I expected him to keep his nose pointed toward the corner. All of these commands were directed toward teaching him self-control. If he violated any of these expectations, I added fifteen seconds to the time.

In the beginning, I had to stand there and ensure he followed through with my instructions. It wasn't always easy, but we found that this form of discipline truly affected him more than anything else we tried.

Don't be afraid to get creative.

Why? Because of his temperament; he was always very active, and sitting still for no other reason than because we told him to directly affected his strong, yet still-carnal, will. Within a matter of weeks, we were beginning to deal with a different little boy. He gradually became more cooperative and began to understand that he didn't always get to do what he wanted.

Don't be afraid to get creative. Talk with other parents about their ideas. Don't be swayed by your children's dismay at being punished or the pressure they may feel at the time you discipline them. They will learn to handle it when they also get all the love and support they need.

A Word About the Rod of Correction

As a society, we have been debating whether or not to spank our children for years now, and the debate seems hotter than ever. While I do believe this form of discipline has often been overused, I don't think we can throw the proverbial baby out with the bath water.

First of all, the Word of God specifically mentions using the "rod of correction" as a form of discipline. Let's briefly look at a couple of these Scriptures. Proverbs 13:24 (NKJV) says, *"He who spares his rod hates his son, but he who loves him disciplines him promptly."* Proverbs 22:15 says, *"Folly is bound up in the heart of a child, but the rod of discipline will drive it far from him."* Proverbs 23:13,14 says, *"Do not withhold discipline from a child; if you punish him with the rod, he will not die. Punish him with the rod and save his soul from death."*

Let's start by defining the word *rod*. It is derived from the Hebrew word *shebet* (pronounced *shay'bet*), and in Scriptures dealing with discipline or rebuke is defined as "a stick for punishing."

Many have attempted to use this word interchangeably with the word *staff*, but this is an entirely different word and meaning. *Staff* is the Hebrew word *mish'-enah* (pronounced *mish-ay-naw'*) and means "support, protection, or sustenance." If we look at Psalm chapter 23, we see both used simultaneously. In verse 4 we see that both the rod (*she'bet*) and staff (*mish'-enah*) bring comfort. Discipline and support bring comfort.

Applying this understanding and definition, we can see that Proverbs 22:15 is telling us that "a stick for punishing" will drive folly out of the hearts of our children. And yes, it really is talking about striking them with that rod of correction. Having established this understanding, let me also say that this form of discipline must be used *carefully* to ensure its effectiveness and protect against physical or emotional harm to your child (abuse).

Remember love must be the number one motivation for any discipline. We discipline because we love our children and have their best interest and future at heart.

We never discipline solely because we are angry or embarrassed. This is especially important when using the "rod" of discipline. Parents must always be in full control of their emotions and actions before spanking their children. By establishing this as a rule for themselves, they are able to prevent abuse by hitting too hard or using an inappropriate tool.

The purpose of swatting a child's behind is not to cause him severe physical pain but to draw his attention in a strong way to the inappropriateness of his actions. It is also not to humiliate him publicly. I personally don't think it is fitting to spank a child in the presence of strangers or even other family members. Children will often be so distracted by the fact that they are embarrassed, they will lose your intended purpose for disciplining them. Keep your motivation and purpose in mind at all times when disciplining. It is a good idea to save this form of discipline for the most severe infractions. Determine ahead of time what offenses are serious enough for this kind of discipline.

For instance, in our home there were three things that would almost always get a spanking: willful disrespect, willful disobedience, and blatant deceit. When someone willfully chooses to do something he knows is wrong, he has violated his own conscience. This is serious business, since it is the root of being self-governed and self-disciplined. You should address this kind of thing immediately and strongly.

All parents must determine what is serious enough for them to use spanking as a discipline and whether or not it will be the most effective for the offense at hand. As in the story about our son and his corner, we had tried spanking—to no avail. Sure, he disliked the swat and even shed a few tears, but he was soon off and running again with no change of heart. The corner, on the other hand, was very effective.

When you do choose to use spanking as a form of discipline, please keep some things in mind: remember to take the child to a private place, be sure he understands why he is being punished, and remind him of the importance of taking responsibility for his choices.

There is really no reason for more than two or three swats—and you should absolutely never leave marks on your child. Teach your children to stand still to receive their punishment or discipline properly and to ensure their safety. I also strongly advise that you apply the "rod" on their behind only!

Reassure your children that you love them and quickly pray with them to help them ask for forgiveness and to learn to listen to the Holy Spirit's leading. Never

We are raising disciples of the Kingdom of God!

bring it up again, just for the sake of bringing it up. Once the offense has been dealt with and forgiven, it is over; Grandma and Aunt Mary don't need to hear about it at the next family get-together. If they repeat the offense and you have to address it again, use the previous examples as points of reference but not as condemnation.

If you apply discipline properly, it will be effective and will produce disciples. Disciples are simply people that follow a particular way with discipline. People who have learned to be disciplined followers (disciples) will also become followers of Christ, believers, participants in the Kingdom of God, supporters and devotees to the principles of the Kingdom, and students and scholars of the Word of God. We are not just training nice, productive members of *this world's* society; we are raising disciples of the *Kingdom of God!*

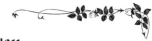

Chapter Eleven

Teaching Your Children the Word of God

2 Timothy 3:14-17 says,

But as for you, continue in what you have learned and have become convinced of, because you know those from whom you learned it, and how from infancy you have known the holy Scriptures, which are able to make you wise for salvation through faith in Christ Jesus. All Scripture is God-breathed and is useful for teaching, rebuking, correcting and training in righteousness, so that the man of God may be thoroughly equipped for every good work.

The life we lead in front of our children is the foundation upon which all of our training and teaching stands. If we live our life after the ideas or standards of the world alone so will our children. On the other hand if the cornerstone of our life is Jesus Christ, the Word of God, our children will follow our example and live their lives after the Word of God as well.

The Word of God is more than mere words or good ideas. It is more than another ancient philosophy. It is alive, active, and powerful (Hebrews 4:12). Paul in verse 16 reminded Timothy that all Scripture is given through the inspiration of God and should be used in every aspect of life (2 Timothy 3:16,17).

As parents, we must live and order our lives by the Word of God first. Matthew tells us to *"seek first his kingdom and his righteousness, and all these things will be given to you as well."* It is the Word of God that is able to penetrate our flesh and directly empower our spirit. Empowerment by the Word of God coupled with that of the Holy Spirit enables us to teach, train, correct, and rebuke our children in righteousness.

Even in the Old Testament, before the Word became flesh and lived among man (John 1:14), David wrote of his dependency on the Word of God.

> *How can a young man keep his way pure? By living according to your word. I seek you with all my heart; do not let me stray from your commands. I have hidden your word in my heart that I might not sin against you. Praise be to you, O LORD; teach me your decrees. With my lips I recount all the laws that come from your mouth. I rejoice in following your statutes as one rejoices in great riches. I meditate on your precepts and consider your ways. I delight in your decrees; I will not neglect your word.*
>
> Psalm 119:9-16

Time after time throughout Psalms, we read psalms about reliance on the decrees, commands, and laws of God. The book of Psalms even begins with the premise that the truly blessed man is one who walks after and delights in the law of the Lord.

It is important that we teach our children to honor and trust in the Word of God. The ways of God are perfect and His word to us is without flaw (Psalm 18:30). Teach your children to understand and then apply the

Word of God in their everyday lives. It is not enough to just hear the Word; you must teach them to *obey* the Word (James 1:22-25).

If your children are arguing beyond reasonable limits, sit them down and teach them what the Word has to say about arguments that bring no true resolution (2 Timothy 3:22-24; Titus 3:9) and how they can be avoided (Proverbs 15:1; 17:14). If your children are becoming anxious and worrying about something, teach them 1 Peter 5:7: *"Cast all your anxiety on him because he cares for you."* Explain to them that our father God is ready, able, and willing to carry and deal with the cares of this world, which so often seem overwhelming to us.

Our children need to have revelations and demonstrations of the power of the Word of God in their daily lives. Remember, the war we fight in the Kingdom of God is not one of flesh and blood, but a spiritual war (Ephesians 6:10-18). Therefore, we don't attempt to fight our battles with fleshly weapons but with our spiritual armor.

For instance, if your children have diligently applied themselves to their schoolwork and still struggle with failure, fight that failure with the Word of God. Attach your faith to Scriptures such as Jeremiah 29:11,12, Jeremiah 33:3, Isaiah 54:13,17, Philippians 4:13, John 15:7,8 and countless others. We want our children to have the same mind-set as Paul did when, even though imprisoned and chained, he knew that would not stop the Word of God from working (2 Timothy 2:9). It may feel to us as if we are chained or that the circumstances of life are working against us, but the Word of God is never chained. It will always continue to live and work in our behalf if we continue in a spirit of faith; it will accomplish what God sends it to accomplish (Isaiah 55:11).

As a revelation of the importance and power of the Word of God begins to grow in our children, so will their desire for it. They will begin through both action and speech to teach and admonish others in the Word of God (Colossians 3:16, 2 Timothy 2:15). The Word of God will begin to produce fruit first in their life and then overflow in the lives of the people with whom they come in contact.

How and Where to Begin

First, the Word of God will bring conviction when needed when you present it to your child with faith and a right spirit. The Holy Spirit knows how to deal with the hearts of our children better than we do. Let Him do His work. If you attempt to do the work of the Holy Spirit, it will only bring condemnation. The result of condemnation is resentment, rebellion, and feelings of guilt and shame. Conviction by the Holy Spirit will result in repentance and a change of heart. Don't use the Word of God to berate your children.

> *The Holy Spirit knows how to deal with the hearts of our children better than we do.*

Memorization

If you look at Psalm 119:9-16 you will see seven ways we can activate the Word of God in our lives.

1. Live (vs. 9)
2. Seek (vs. 10)
3. Hide (vs. 11)
4. Recount (vs. 13)
5. Rejoice (vs. 14)
6. Meditate (vs. 15)
7. Delight/not neglect (vs. 16)

By memorizing the Word of God, we are able to activate any of the above seven at any time. Be careful that you are not only teaching your children the words but also the spirit and revelation of the Word.

For example, one of the Scriptures I taught our children is 2 Chronicles 34:3. The Scripture talks about a young king of Judah, Josiah, who began to reign when he was only eight years old. It says while he was still young, he began to seek the God of his father David. The point of telling them this story was to help them understand the importance of beginning to seek God while they were young. Rather than just memorize the third verse, we also talked about the whole story of Josiah's reign. It made the significance of his beginning to serve God at a young age relevant to them.

We had been working on memorizing 1 Peter 5:7, *"Cast all your cares on him for he cares for you."* Our son had come up with the idea to pretend as though he were casting a fishing pole in order to remember the word *cast*. Our daughter decided to pretend to rock a baby in her arms to remember the phrase, *"he cares for you."*

It was working for them, but while they could remember the verse, they were having trouble recalling the exact chapter and verse. They would get stuck after 1 Peter, and then they drew a blank. So one day as we began to recite the verse, when they reached the end and said 1 Peter..., I shouted "five seven!" Both of them broke into fits of laughter because I had startled them, which was my intention. They never forgot the chapter and verse again! Each time we recited that verse, we all shouted out "five seven!" from then on.

Use every tool available to you to help your children memorize Scripture. Search out videos and music tapes or CDs that put Scripture to music or some sort of cadence. Use actions and pictures to represent words.

Involve your children in coming up with the actions or pictures so that it really means something to them.

Using pictures to represent words is an excellent way to help your children memorize Scriptures. Creating a picture to represent a word is called a rebus, and our children—with some assistance—have created many such pictures to help their memorization process and even drew most of them themselves!

So we had three things helping them to memorize: the verbal repetition, their own creativity, and the actual drawing of each picture. They were not only hearing the Scripture, they were doing something with it to help store it in their memory.

We have used all sorts of games, books, puzzles, even flashcards I found at a local dollar store to help teach and reinforce memorization. Always be on the look out for things your children would find enjoyable aids in learning. Don't give them word puzzles if they don't enjoy words puzzles. Let them act out a Scripture (a sort of charades type game) if they enjoy that. Nearly all children benefit from putting any kind of new information to music. Scripture set to music is readily available to parents at Christian bookstores and even in some regular discount department stores. There are also some incredible board games, videos, and books available. There are even video games that reinforce Scripture memorization!

Don't feel overwhelmed by the idea of memorizing Scripture with your children. Keep in mind, it is not necessarily about the quantity you are able to memorize but the fact that you are establishing a habit of memorizing the Word of God. Try to schedule a regular time to work on Scripture reading and memorization. Be consistent to the best of your ability. Don't feel pressure for it to take a great length of time, either. The younger your children are, the shorter the time span should be.

When our children were infants, each night as we put them to bed we would speak the Word of God over them and pray as part of our bedtime routine. As they grew older, we involved them in the routine. We had a small booklet that had good Scripture confessions in it. It wasn't always the exact Scripture; they were often a paraphrased version that emphasized the context of it. One of our daughter's favorites was, "No one can take my joy away. Jesus is my joy!" (from John 16:22) Our son's favorite was, "God is the strength of my life. I can do anything with Jesus in me!" (from Philippians 4:13) This is one of his favorite Scriptures to this day!

It wasn't the amount of time we spent with them that taught them these truths but the fact that we were consistent with it. We used that little confession book for years. It still sits on a bookshelf in my office.

When to Start

When your children are infants, begin with something simple. Begin even before your children fully comprehend what you are saying or doing—while your child is still in the womb is good! The sooner you begin to establish a routine, the better off you are.

As your children age and mature, teach Scriptures that coincide with holidays, teach character, are relevant to a particular situation they are working through, or Scriptures that center on a particular theme such as prayer or salvation.

Below you will find some ideas and recommendations.

Holidays

Christmas
- Luke 2—story of Jesus' birth
- 2 Corinthians 8 & 9, Proverbs 11:24,25—giving

Valentine's Day
- 1 Corinthians 13—love defined
- John 3:16—love demonstrated
- Matthew 22:37-40—love commanded

The Fourth of July
- Romans 8—freedom from sin and death
- Galatians 5—set free, don't become bound again

Themes

Prayer
- Matthew 6:5-13—Jesus' teaching on prayer, Lord's prayer
- Mark 11:24, Luke 6:28—praying for forgiveness and being thankful

Thankfulness/Gratitude
- Psalm 100:4, Psalm 136:1, Colossians 3:17—being thankful
- Luke 17:11-19—story of ten lepers
- 1 Thessalonians 5:17, James 5:13—praying and being thankful

Contentment
- Hebrews 13:5, 1 Timothy 6:6—godliness with contentment is gain

Other examples of themes might include forgiveness, salvation, work of Holy Spirit, sharing your faith, and cheerfulness.

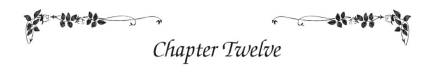

Chapter Twelve

Fearfully and Wonderfully Made

Some people mistakenly confuse temperament and personality with character. Your children's temperament or personality is their individual identity, their natural disposition, and the particulars of the way they see the world. This is different than character: children are born with their own unique personalities, but you as the parent must teach them character. You can help your children by asking God for revelation about their personality—the way they are going to go—but you have a responsibility to help them develop a moral compass and the ability to distinguish right from wrong.

> *Children are born with their own unique personalities, but you as the parent must teach them character.*

Earlier in this book, we looked at Psalm 139:13-16 and the words *fearfully* and *wonderfully.*

> *For you created my inmost being; you knit me together in my mother's womb. I praise you because I am fearfully and wonderfully made; your works are wonderful, I know that full well.*

This passage conveys to us the great care God took in creating human beings.

It is easy to look around at the people we know and see certain characteristics about them that set them apart from others. As we look at the lives of many of the people of the Bible, it's easy to see that God creates everything with purpose in mind. Peter was sometimes rash or aggressive in his thinking and behavior, but it was that aggressiveness and boldness that caused him to stand and boldly declare the gospel on the day of Pentecost. Three thousand people's lives were changed that day because of his boldness. David's deep emotions and passion in his psalms have helped us to worship God. How often have you been unable to find the words you wanted to say to God only to come across one of David's psalms reflecting your heart?

Nothing God creates is by accident or without purpose. Revelation 4:11 says, *"You are worthy, our Lord and God, to receive glory and honor and power: for you created all things, and by your will they were created and have their being."*

Ultimately, who and what we are is for the purpose of God and His Kingdom. As parents, we must consider the type of personality and temperament our children have when teaching and training them.

I think God chose Peter because he was a bit impetuous and hotheaded at times. He didn't let Peter stay that way, though. He worked with him and taught him how to make his temperament work for him, and in the end, we see miraculous results and fruit in his life. You are not aiming to recreate your children in a new image that you fancy; parents are to train children so their temperament helps them in their calling.

Begin by doing a little research into basic personality and temperament types. There are many excellent books available that address these topics and that are specifically geared toward helping you spot your children's character type early. Many of the authors of these books also hold workshops for families. The knowledge you gain will help you to begin to identify and understand your child's temperament—and maybe your own as well!

Let's say you are a more extroverted-type personality—you like to be the life of the party and meet new people. Your child, on the other hand, is more reserved, introverted, and loves to quietly read and write poetry. How do you think these differences could affect your relationship? For one thing, when you attend a party together some of your antics may embarrass her, and her lack of socializing may frustrate you. "Why won't she just get out there and meet some people?" you might wonder. Meanwhile, she's probably wondering why you must always be so loud and obnoxious! Neither temperament is *wrong*; they're just different. But hopefully from this example you can begin to see how understanding temperaments might help you in your relationship with your children.

Temperament differences will affect the way you teach and discipline your children as well. You'll have a lot of conflict potential if you are a parent that's a strong leader and organizer but your child is a spontaneous free-spirit. You'll probably be constantly trying to get your child to be more organized, and he'll probably have trouble understanding the point. There's a good chance he *needs* to be more organized, but if you understand his temperament, you'll be able to use wisdom in helping him see the need for orderliness and schedules. He may never be similar to you, but his free-spirit nature is what makes him unique! Too much control and organization will stifle his creativity, so it's up to you to help find balance in your teaching.

There are many differences in people, and understanding these differences will go a long way in helping to resolve conflicts in your family relationships. People might fit into different broad personality types, and you might be able to get some understanding through research and paying attention, but each of your children are unique. Your most reliable source for information on them will always be their Father in heaven, who created both of you!

Some Final Thoughts

Thought #1

Being a parent is *fun*! When we parents relax and stop worrying about jobs, dishes, or even the unpaid bills for a while, you'll find your children can be quite entertaining and amusing. I have heard some of the funniest and craziest stories from fellow parents.

My brother, at the wonderful age of six years, told our dear sweet neighbor lady she had a fat behind—I believe his exact words were, "Mable, you have a fat butt." My mother nearly passed out right there in the middle of the yard while my brother and I staggered around laughing hysterically. Our practical neighbor told my mother she should never punish my brother for speaking the truth. Yeah right! We were both in hot water.

Here's another good one on my brother. He used to love to hide and jump out and scare my mother. Her reactions were just too fun to resist. One evening we were all settling in to watch television together, and our mother went to make popcorn. As she emerged from the kitchen, huge bowl of popcorn in hand, he jumped out from behind the piano and yelled. She, predictably, screamed and, unpredictably, threw the whole bowl of popcorn straight up into the air. We were discovering popcorn kernels under furniture for days.

A friend of mine has four boys. Her two oldest are close to our son's age, and they spend quite a bit of time together. One day a few years ago they were all at her house playing outside near a small creek and discovered it had fish in it. So they caught one and brought it into the house for my friend to cook for dinner. Couple of problems here—first, no one would dare eat anything out of that creek, and second, the fish had been dead for quite some time and it looked as if some other critter had already had it for dinner. Her shrieks of horror did nothing to discourage their assertion that there was still some good meat on those bones and that they could fillet it off if she'd just give them a knife. Thank goodness they were at her house and not mine!

There is nothing funnier or more exciting than watching children explore and discover their world.

Have fun with your children—create it if you have to. Our children used to have the most intense games of indoor hide-and-seek with their father you could ever dream of. I'm still amazed at the places they all found to hide.

Look at these moments and find the humor in them. There is nothing funnier or more exciting than watching children explore and discover their world as they grow into adulthood.

Thought #2

If while reading this book you've realized there are some things you should do differently, don't be discouraged. There is not one perfect parent on the planet. Every one of us needs work in some area. Write down what you would like to change and how you can begin to make those changes.

One of the biggest changes I had to make was teaching my children to obey me the first time. I sat my children down and told them it was important for them to learn to obey their parents the first time we ask them to do something. I explained that we were going to begin to expect that of them and if they did not obey the first time there would be consequences (I didn't use that word though, they were young). For the next week, each time they were told or asked to do something and they did not move the first time, we reminded them that beginning next week there would be consequences. We kept our word.

It wasn't always easy to follow through. It was a process. We had to make a decision and not turn back. Step by step, little by little, we saw results. We saw results in us and in our children.

Thought #3

I have five simple keys I'd like you to keep in mind. I call them The Five Parenting Keys. How's that for creativity?

1. Prayer – Begin here and don't stop. I am convinced that this is the greatest source of strength and help for every parent.
2. Love – Your children need, crave and deserve your unconditional, unending love. If you need to, reread chapter four. Your love should be the number one motivating factor for encouraging and disciplining your children.
3. Acceptance – This goes hand in hand with love. Accept and celebrate who God made your children to be. Train them, mold their temperament and personalities, but don't attempt to change them.
4. Time – Time really is of the essence when it comes to kids. Spend as much time with them as you can. I've heard some say quality is better than quantity. I think a quantity of quality time with your children is best. You cannot impart to

them if you are not spending time with them. Make time with your children a priority. Take them to the park, ice cream stand, or the zoo. Spend time messing around in the backyard, talking with them and listening, listening, listening (get the point?) to them. You can't beat a good old-fashioned family dinner with everyone seated at a table and looking at each other.

I realize that many families today have experienced divorce or other circumstances that prevent them from physically spending the amount of time they would like with their children.

Let me ask you this. Where is your heart? When your children are with you, are you distracted by other things or are you making them a priority? When they are not with you, do you telephone or send them cards or notes to let them know you are thinking of them? There are ways that we can give our children our time even when they are not physically with us.

5. Discipline – I don't need to elaborate much on this as I've written a whole chapter on this as well. Just one small point—of the five keys, I listed this one last on purpose. I want to remind us that the first four lay the groundwork for this one. It is vitally important that we discipline our children and just as important that we pray, love, accept, and spend time with them. Remember to keep the scale balanced.

I'm a list maker so I wrote these out and put them somewhere to help keep me focused. You may not want or need to write them out. The five keys are meant to be highlights or quick reminders of what should be priorities for parents. If I had two minutes to talk with a parent these are the five things I would tell them.

My Final Thought

Being a parent is one of the most challenging, exciting, rewarding endeavors any individual could undertake. It is a journey like no other journey, and unfortunately there is not a precise road map to follow. Interestingly, God said he orders the steps of a righteous man. He also said that His Word would light our path and that the path of the righteous gets brighter and brighter until it is fully lit and easily seen. This is how parenting is. When a child comes into our lives our steps have been ordered for the next eighteen years and beyond. Yet often we find ourselves not knowing which direction to take. It is the Word of God that shines light on those steps, and the more we look to God and His Word for answers the brighter the steps ahead become until we are clear which direction we should take.

My goal in this book is not to write an exhaustive reference book or lexicon with all the answers for every parenting moment. I don't believe that is humanly possible. What parent would have time to read it anyway? My goal is to inspire you and give you hope. Don't worry about the past—look to the well-lit path of your future and remember God is your source.

Author Contact Information

Kathi Pitts

Cornerstone Church

P.O. Box 351690

Toledo, OH 43635

www.cornerstonechurch.us

The Five Parenting Keys

1. Prayer

2. Love

3. Acceptance

4. Time

5. Discipline

Notes

Notes

Books by Michael Pitts

Don't Curse Your Crisis

Breaking Ungodly Soul Ties

Help! I Think God is Trying to Kill Me

Breaking the Assignment of Spiritual Assassins

A Dictionary of Contemporary Words and Concepts

Making the Holy Spirit Your Partner

Living on the Edge

To purchase books, tape series, videos, and other product materials by Michael Pitts please visit our web site at www.cornerstonechurch.us